the Unofficial Guide™ to Overcoming Arthritis

Lisa Iannucci
with
Mark Horowitz, M.D.

Macmillan • USA

Macmillan General Reference USA
A Pearson Education Macmillan Company
1633 Broadway
New York, New York 10019-6785

ISBN: 0-02862714-8

Manufactured in the United States of America

10 9 8 7 6 5 4 3 2 1

First edition

This book is dedicated to my mother, Patricia Quaglieri, who had faith in me since I was a child, and who taught me that I had the strength and perseverance to overcome any obstacles in my way. My mother is an inspiration, and I appreciate her for the dedication and love she has given to her family. Thank you, Mom, for loving me, believing in me, and teaching me to believe in myself.

Acknowledgments

My heartfelt thanks to my husband, Jeff Brinkley, and my children, Nicole, Travis, and Samantha, for their understanding and patience throughout this project. Jeff, thank you for making me hot chocolate late at night, researching material on the Internet, and the hundreds of other ways you supported me. Thanks especially for your encouragement—you helped make this book happen. And thanks also to my children, who drew pictures to cheer me up when I was working late—you are my inspiration.

Thanks also to my development editor, Nancy Gratton—I am extremely grateful for your devotion to this project, and your secure belief in my abilities. You helped me to stay focused and inspired me to see this book through. I will never forget your support and hard work to make this book a reality.

Thanks to Mark Horowitz, M.D., for your guidance and the expertise you provided on the more strictly medical aspects of this book. Thanks also to the staff at the Grinnell Library in Wappingers Falls, New York, especially to the librarians who pitched in with their exceptional researching skills and endless patience for my (sometimes last-minute) requests.

Finally, thanks to the good people at Alpha Books: Kathy Niebenhaus, publisher; Jennifer Perillo, managing editor; Scott Barnes, production editor; and Bette LaGow, copyeditor.

Contents

The *Unofficial Guide* Reader's Bill of Rights

We Give You More Than the Official Line

Welcome to the *Unofficial Guide* series of Lifestyles titles—books that deliver critical, unbiased information that other books can't or won't reveal—*the inside scoop*. Our goal is to provide you with the *most accessible, useful* information and advice possible. The recommendations we offer in these pages are not influenced by the corporate line of any organization or industry; we give you the hard facts, whether those institutions like them or not. If something is ill-advised or will cause a loss of time and/or money, we'll give you ample warning. And if it is a worthwhile option, we'll let you know that, too.

Armed and Ready

Our hand-picked authors confidently and critically report on a wide range of topics that matter to smart readers like you. Our authors are passionate about their subjects, but have distanced themselves enough from them to help you be armed and protected, and help you make educated decisions as you go through your process. It is our intent that, from having read this book, you will avoid the pitfalls everyone else falls into and get it right the first time.

Don't be fooled by cheap imitations; this is the *genuine article Unofficial Guide* series from Macmillan Publishing. You may be familiar with our proven track record of the travel *Unofficial Guides*, which have more than three million copies in print. Each year thousands of travelers—new and old—are armed with a brand new, fully updated edition of the flagship *Unofficial Guide to Walt Disney World*, by Bob Sehlinger. It is our intention here to provide you with the same level of objective authority that Mr. Sehlinger does in his brainchild.

The Unofficial Panel of Experts

Every work in the Lifestyle *Unofficial Guides* is intensively inspected by a team of top professionals in their fields. These experts review the manuscript for factual accuracy, comprehensiveness, and an insider's determination as to whether the manuscript fulfills the credo in this Reader's Bill of Rights. In other words, our Panel ensures that you are, in fact, getting "the inside scoop."

Our Pledge

The authors, the editorial staff, and the Unofficial Panel of Experts assembled for *Unofficial Guides* are determined to lay out the most valuable alternatives available for our readers. This dictum means that our writers must be explicit, prescriptive, and above all, direct. We strive to be thorough and complete, but our goal is not necessarily to have the "most" or "all" of the information on a topic; this is not, after all, an encyclopedia. Our objective is to help you narrow down your options to the best of what is available, unbiased by affiliation with any industry or organization.

In each *Unofficial Guide* we give you:

- Comprehensive coverage of necessary and vital information
- Authoritative, rigidly fact-checked data
- The most up-to-date insights into trends
- Savvy, sophisticated writing that's also readable
- Sensible, applicable facts and secrets that only an insider knows

Special Features

Every book in our series offers the following six special sidebars in the margins that were devised to help you get things done cheaply, efficiently, and smartly.

1. "Timesaver"—tips and shortcuts that save you time.
2. "Moneysaver"—tips and shortcuts that save you money.
3. "Watch Out!"—more serious cautions and warnings.
4. "Bright Idea"—general tips and shortcuts to help you find an easier or smarter way to do something.
5. "Quote"—statements from real people that are intended to be prescriptive and valuable to you.
6. "Unofficially..."—an insider's fact or anecdote.

We also recognize your need to have quick information at your fingertips, and have thus provided the following comprehensive sections at the back of the book:

1. **Glossary:** Definitions of complicated terminology and jargon.

2. **Resource Guide:** Lists of relevant agencies, associations, institutions, web sites, etc.

3. **Recommended Reading List:** Suggested titles that can help you get more in-depth information on related topics.

4. **Index.**

Letters, Comments, and Questions from Readers

We strive to continually improve the Unofficial series, and input from our readers is a valuable way for us to do that. Many of those who have used the *Unofficial Guide* travel books write to the authors to ask questions, make comments, or share their own discoveries and lessons. For lifestyle *Unofficial Guides*, we would also appreciate all such correspondence, both positive and critical, and we will make best efforts to incorporate appropriate readers' feedback and comments in revised editions of this work.

How to write to us:

Unofficial Guides
Macmillan Lifestyle Guides
Macmillan Publishing
1633 Broadway
New York, NY 10019

Attention: Reader's Comments

The *Unofficial Guide* Panel of Experts

The *Unofficial* editorial team recognizes that you've purchased this book with the expectation of getting the most authoritative, carefully inspected information currently available. Toward that end, on each and every title in this series, we have selected a minimum of two "official" experts comprising the "Unofficial Panel" who painstakingly review the manuscripts to ensure: factual accuracy of all data; inclusion of the most up-to-date and relevant information; and that, from an insider's perspective, the authors have armed you with all the necessary facts you need—but the institutions don't want you to know.

For *The Unofficial Guide to Overcoming Arthritis,* we are proud to introduce the following panel of experts:

Dedee Benrey is a certified yoga instructor with extensive experience in creating natural lifestyles. She teaches yoga and healing-arts workshops in health clubs and spas around the U.S. Her innovative seminars and yoga workshops are regularly offered at the New York

Health and Racquet Clubs, Chelsea Piers, and the prestigious New York Open Center.

Maureen M. McSweeney, Ph.D., is a psychologist who specializes in pain management and stress reduction. A member of the American Pain Society and other professional organizations, she serves on the Patient Services Committee for the New York chapter of the Arthritis Foundation. She has been featured on *Good Morning America* as a spokesperson for the Arthritis Foundation regarding the use of T'ai Chi and Qi Dong for people with arthritis.

Introduction

Imagine that this introduction was written in French, Greek, or Latin—or any other language that is foreign to you. To understand it, you would need an interpreter; someone to explain all the unfamiliar words.

This is probably how you feel when you pour over medical research, books, articles, or Internet pages eager for answers to your questions about arthritis. The bottom line is that medical research is mostly written for doctors, not patients. You need someone to translate that medical research into a language that you can understand.

On the subject of arthritis, this book is your translator. *The Unofficial Guide to Overcoming Arthritis* has been written in no-nonsense, matter-of-fact language so that you can understand your condition, identify the treatments available to you, know what questions to ask your physician, and learn how to live, work, and survive with arthritis.

Think back: as a child were you taught, probably in an elementary school health class or by your parents, to "take care of your body if you want to grow up to be healthy?" It was good advice, but good health is a concept that you probably did not pay much attention to until you were sick. Then you felt guilty that you didn't pay as close attention to your health as you should have when you were younger. You reflected on what you could have done to keep your body healthier.

Forget the guilt; you can better your body at any age. Medical science is beginning to prove that some forms of arthritis are inborn; you are going to get it no matter what you do. Instead of dwelling on what you could have or should have done, you should be arming yourself with the information that will help you now, no matter what type of arthritis you have, or whether you are in active pain or remission.

To start the process, Part One, "The Hard Facts About Arthritis," will educate you on your body, specifically your musculoskeletal system—your bones, muscles, and tissues. You will learn about the development of your bones and how they change as you age. You will learn what you can do to strengthen the bones, such as eating right and exercising.

One of the most important factors in successfully treating and managing your pain is to have it diagnosed as soon as possible. Pain is your body's way of signaling to you that there is something wrong, and it should never be ignored. There are many specialized tests to help diagnose your pain, from blood work to specialized genetic testing that determines if you are genetically susceptible to getting a particular form of arthritis. Knowing what these tests are is an important step in understanding the results and living with them.

Once you are done with Part One you will have a basic understanding of your body, how arthritis affects your body, and the medical tests that are used to diagnose your arthritis.

Part Two, "Types of Arthritis," will first give you an in-depth easy-to-understand look at two of the most common forms of arthritis: osteoarthritis and rheumatoid arthritis; conditions that affect over 17 million Americans combined, including 285,000 children.

The past two decades were marked by better recognition of fibromyalgia, a muscle and joint syndrome that affects millions of Americans. Fibromyalgia isn't arthritis, but it mimics it and has often been misdiagnosed as arthritis. I found it vital to focus on this condition in an entire chapter, since many patients who are struggling to be diagnosed will probably look to books on arthritis for the answers.

There are over 100 types of arthritis, and each one could fill an entire book on its own, so it is impossible to discuss each one here in detail. The final section of part two will give you a rundown of other types of arthritis, such as ankylosing spondylitis, Lyme disease, scleroderma and gout.

In Part Three, "Treatment and Medication," I separate fact from fiction. Arthritis patients are desperate for answers, and desperate for relief of their pain. Some patients may believe any snake oil salesperson trying to sell them a concoction of "cures" for their pain. Chapter 8 dispels many of these so-called cures, and helps you to recognize quack products; this chapter may save you before you subject yourself to a dangerous product.

Chapter 9 is about medication to alleviate your symptoms; it is not about cures. Today, however, there are a great variety of medications for your physicians to choose from and prescribe to help alleviate your symptoms. Only a few decades ago, arthritis sufferers relied on aspirin to reduce the pain and inflammation, but today there are hundreds of options. The medical industry has made great strides in the past decades by introducing new medications, and it is important to understand how this medication will affect you and treat your arthritis, and how to take it safely.

Good health means good nutrition, exercise, and taking care of you by minimizing stress. Millions of Americans each year make New Year's resolutions to lose weight and get in shape, or to take better care of their bodies. It is estimated that by the third week of January, most New Year's resolutions have already been broken. Why? Because most Americans do not understand how to eat right and exercise right.

Eating well and exercising have tremendous amounts of health benefits and, in turn, your bones and joints benefit from a healthier body. Chapters 12 and 13 will show you how exercise and nutrition affect your arthritis and how you can exercise and eat right.

Millions of Americans are turning to alternative therapies, such as herbs, magnets, chiropractors, and acupuncture to treat their illnesses. Patients who suffer from arthritis may also use alternative treatments to help ease other symptoms, such as headaches that have been caused by the stress of having a chronic illness, or dry skin caused by medications. Although the medical community has been hesitant to approve these treatments for arthritis unless there are scientific studies that prove their effectiveness and safety, it is important to recognize that these treatments are being used and understand how they affect your arthritis and your overall health.

Surgery is not a last resort, and chapter 10 will explain how surgery can bring long-awaited relief to your suffering, especially artificial joint replacement surgery. Before you jump in and agree to any procedures, there are many factors to consider. It is important to understand what the risks of surgery are and the length and complexity of the recovery process.

How do you handle it all? Check out Chapters 14 and 15 in Part Four, "Lifestyle Changes to Ease Arthritis," to learn how you can handle the pain of your arthritis in your daily life. It is not a smooth road all of the time and many who suffer from arthritis will tell you that there are ups and downs. Arthritis can affect your job, your family and your sex life. You may need to talk to others who have been in the same position as you are in now. Support groups are there for you. When you need to talk, or just want to listen to others who have experienced the same feelings that you have, support groups can help. Finding one that works for you is important, whether it is a group, online chat room, or individual counseling.

Incidentally, I brought to the writing of this book my own personal understanding of the importance of overcoming arthritis. I have long been aware of that I am susceptible to the condition in my knees. And while writing this book I was myself on a diagnostic quest to learn what was causing me frequent, debilitating pain. The diagnosis was that I had myofascial pain, a form of fibromyalgia (see Chapter 5).

The good news is that for both conditions, writing this book has given me more power and understanding about my body and health than I had before. And most of all, it has allowed me to share the hope and help available to all who suffer from the disease known as arthritis. We may not yet have a cure for arthritis, but we can certainly find ways to keep ourselves vital and active, in spite of it.

The Hard Facts About Arthritis

GET THE SCOOP ON...
Arthritis and you ▪ Bones and aging ▪
The causes of arthritis ▪ Symptoms to watch for

PART I

Bone Breakdown: What Is Arthritis?

W hen you are healthy, you probably take your body for granted. It's usually only when it breaks down—whether due to an accident, illness, disease, or everyday wear and tear—that you recognize the importance of good health and your body's extraordinary capabilities to heal and repair itself.

For optimum health, you should have a basic understanding of how your body works and feels when you are well, not just when you are injured or sick. No one expects you to have the knowledge of a medical professional about the human anatomy, but a basic understanding can help you recognize if something is wrong with your body and help you explain any aches, pains, and abnormalities to your doctor.

For example, if you are in the habit of performing regular monthly breast exams, you understand what your breasts normally look and feel like. You would be quick to notice any abnormalities, such as

3

Unofficially...
Arthritis and gout were well known during the Byzantine Empire (324-1453 AD). Fourteen of 86 Byzantine emperors may have been afflicted with gout or arthritis. At that time, the cause was explained by excessive eating, drinking of alcohol, stress, heredity, and sexual promiscuity.

a lump or swelling, and be able to describe these to your physician. This would be the same for men who are in the habit of performing monthly testicular exams. Armed with this information, your doctor is in a better position to order the necessary tests and prescribe the proper treatment. Without this familiarity and understanding of your own body, you might overlook potential problems or not be in the position to explain a problem adequately to your doctor.

This same familiarity and understanding of your body works in your favor with all aspects of your personal health. If you have been diagnosed with a form of arthritis, you have a chronic condition—this means that once you are diagnosed, you will have it for life. The condition can enter periods of remission, and there are medications that can help to control the pain and inflammation, but almost all forms of arthritis are, at present, incurable. Understanding and becoming familiar with how your own body moves and feels will aid you in monitoring the progress of your condition and help you receive the proper medical treatment when necessary.

This chapter will provide you with the information necessary to gain an understanding of your body. Unfortunately, at our current stage of medical knowledge, this information may not address or answer all of your questions. There have been many advancements regarding arthritis, but it still remains something of a medical mystery. Scientists are still researching its causes and are still experimenting with new treatments. This should not discourage you from using any knowledge you gain to manage your health to the best of your ability.

The life of the bone

To understand how arthritis affects your body, you need to become familiar with your musculoskeletal system, which includes your muscles and bones. The human skeletal system consists of 206 bones. These bones are held together by ligaments—flexible bands of tissue—which are neither muscle nor bone. Bones, ligaments, and muscles provide a framework for the entire body. Simply put, every bone works in conjunction with a muscle. When a muscle contracts, the bones to which it is attached move as well. Just imagine a skeleton hanging in a doorway at Halloween. The skeleton is a limp pile of bones, unable to move without the help of muscles, ligaments, and cartilage. Cartilage is a rubbery substance that protects the bone and reduces the friction between two adjacent bones (say, when they meet each other at a joint like the elbow or the knee) by forming a protective cushion. Tendons attach muscles to bone so they can move in conjunction. All of these components of a joint act as a team to help the joint to move.

This rigid internal structure serves two functions:

1. It allows the body to bend and move.
2. It protects vital organs. For example, the ribcage protects the heart and the skull protects the brain.

The bones in the skeleton are not just an inert frame, however; bones also produce blood cells and store important minerals, such as calcium and phosphorous, until they are needed. Calcium builds bones and helps them remain strong. Calcium also helps muscles to contract, the heart to beat, and blood to clot. Ninety-nine percent of the calcium in

Watch Out!
Do not attempt to diagnose or treat yourself no matter how closely your symptoms resemble any medical condition. This can be dangerous to your health, as symptoms can often be misleading. Have a complete physical performed to rule out any other possible conditions.

your body is stored in your bones and teeth. When your system is in short supply of this necessary mineral, your body takes the stored calcium from the bones, leaving the bones weaker and more prone to injury.

The other mineral stored in your bones, phosphorous, is also major component of bones and teeth, second only to calcium. Phosphorus is used to metabolize the calcium so that your body can use it. But your bones did not start out as bones. Here is a little tour through the development of your skeletal system:

1. In the first few weeks of pregnancy, a tiny embryo already has the beginnings of a skeletal system in the form of tiny limb buds. Later, these buds take the shape of arms, legs, and joints, and by the second trimester—the middle months of pregnancy—these joints and limbs are fully usable.

2. Surprisingly, a newborn has more bones than an adult. At birth, a baby has 350 "bones," which are actually made out of cartilage. As the child grows, this cartilage is replaced by bone; the bones then fuse together to create larger units and eventually the skeleton has 206 adult bones, formed through a process called ossification. These bones continue to lengthen and harden until the child is about 20 years old, at which point the bones are considered fully developed.

If you split a human bone in half and look inside, you might be surprised to find that bones are strong, but not heavy or solid all the way through. Bones are broken down into three layers:

Bright Idea
Mom said, "drink milk, it's good for your bones"—and she was right. Calcium is found in milk products, and (for the lactose intolerant among you) in broccoli, sardines, and salmon. It's never too late to increase your calcium intake. While you can't repair any existing damage by drinking milk, added calcium *can* help to strengthen bones and muscles.

- Periosteum, a outer layer that contains a network of blood vessels and nerves that supply the bones with oxygen and nutrients. The periosteum is thick and rich in young bones, and thinner, with fewer vessels, later in life.

- Compact bone, the next layer, which is a hard dense shell laced with canals that carry blood vessels, lymph, and nerves.

- Cancellous bone, the soft middle layer at the center of the bone, filled with a fatty tissue called marrow that produces red and white blood cells and platelets.

Bones are connected to each other at joints. When you bend, twist, or turn, joints provide the flexibility to move these bones into position. There are three types of joints in the body:

- Free-moving, or synovial joints, such as the knees or elbows, which are highly flexible.

- Part-moving, such as your spine, which allows for more restricted movement.

- Non-moving, firmly fixed joints such as the ones that connect most of the bones in your skull.

Bones are living tissue, not hard, static structures. Every day, old bone is removed and replaced with new bone tissue. Even after your bones have stopped growing in size and length (as discussed above), the density of the bone continues to grow.

Bones continue to increase their density and calcium content until you reach your 30s, at which point you probably have attained your peak bone mass. As you age, you will either maintain this amount of bone mass, or your bones will begin to lose calcium steadily each year. However, you cannot increase the amount of bone density after this point.

Unofficially...
The oldest mummy in the world was discovered in 1991 in the Oetz Valley (now part of Italy). The 5,300-year-old mummy, nicknamed Oetzi, is believed to have died of exhaustion at about age 45. Experts guess he was five feet five and 88 pounds when he died. They believe he suffered from arthritis and that the 57 tattoos on his body were a Neolithic therapy for his condition.

This thinning process occurs more rapidly in women—at a rate of about one percent per year. When a woman goes through menopause, she loses more bone density because her body has stopped producing estrogen, a hormone required to improve bone strength. As both men and women age, any bone loss puts their bones at a higher risk for osteoporosis and arthritis.

As mentioned earlier, in a normal joint where two bones meet, the ends are coated with cartilage "cushion." There is also a fluid between the bones of the joint, called the synovial fluid, which acts as a lubricant. Ligaments surround and support each joint and connect the bones. When all of these elements of a normal joint are present and functioning properly, you can pretty much take for granted your ability for movement. Unfortunately, for people with arthritis, this elegant system does not work as well as it should.

What is arthritis?

Now that you have a better understanding of the musculoskeletal system, the workings of a normal joint, and how your bones age, you can now understand how the system can break down and how that breakdown can affect your bones.

The word "arthritis" comes from two Greek words: arthros, meaning "joint" and the suffix -itis, which means "inflammation." Arthritis is a general term used to describe more than 100 different rheumatic diseases that affect the joints, muscles, and connective tissues of the body. The two most prevalent forms of arthritis are osteoarthritis (OA) and rheumatoid arthritis (RA). Osteoarthritis affects specific joints, whereas rheumatoid arthritis, and other rheumatic diseases, may result in restricted

Unofficially...
In May, 1972, a Presidential Proclamation designated each May as National Arthritis Month to help increase awareness of all forms of arthritis.

movement in all of the joints and tissues. There are many myths surrounding arthritis, including:

- *Everyone gets it as they age.* Although it is estimated that more than 40 million Americans, or one in six people, have been diagnosed with arthritis, that hardly adds up to "everyone." And it is not just a disease associated with aging; it can strike anyone, even infants. Approximately 285,000 children in the United States have juvenile arthritis for which the causes are unknown.

- *Cracking my knuckles will lead to arthritis.* The cracking sound is simply caused by a rapid release of the synovial fluid inside the joint, not by any real damage done directly to the joint. While cracking knuckles is unpleasant to anyone who has to listen to that popping sound, it is nonetheless relatively harmless.

- *If I'm stiff or have joint pain, it means that I have arthritis.* Morning stiffness or pain in your joints does not put you at risk for arthritis, nor does it mean that you already have arthritis. These symptoms can signify other conditions including:

1. Overexercising: exercising too long or too hard can cause muscle soreness, stiffness, and possible pain from a pull or strain.

2. Injury: damage to bones, joints, or muscles caused by injury can leave you with stiffness and soreness for an extended period of time.

3. Soft-tissue damage: conditions such as tennis or golfer's elbow, where a particular motion is performed for a lengthy period of time, can cause inflammation of the tendons in your arm.

These conditions are not arthritis, but are instead the results of injury, strain, or inflammation of the tendons and ligaments. And these conditions do not "turn into" arthritis.

4. Stress: when you are emotionally stressed, you have a tendency to tighten your muscles, which can lead to muscle spasms in the neck and shoulders, lower back pain, and aches in your bones. Stress is indicated as a factor in many illnesses and can also aggravate an existing health problem.

5. Depression: feeling sad and tired are not the only symptoms of depression. Depression can manifest physical symptoms, including headaches, constipation, abdominal problems and aches and pains in your bones.

Clearly, stiffness, pain, and swelling in the joints can be symptoms of many other illnesses and diseases—they do not necessarily indicate arthritis. For this reason, attempting to do your own self-diagnosis is not a good idea. If you are experiencing stiffness, pain, and swelling, it is important that you have yourself examined before jumping to conclusions and causing yourself undue stress.

While most of the beliefs mentioned earlier are relatively harmless, some false assumptions can, in fact, be dangerous. For example, many people believe that arthritis only affects your bones. This is simply not true. In addition to your bones, arthritis can affect the connective tissue—the tissue that holds the muscles, ligaments, tendons, and synovial membranes together. Scleroderma is one member of the arthritis "family" that does just that: It is a disease of the connective tissue that causes a thickening and hardening of the skin. Systemic lupus erythematosus, also known as lupus, is another serious disorder classed under the name of arthritis that can inflame and damage not only the joints, but other connective tissues of the body.

Arthritis can also be fatal. Rheumatoid arthritis, for example, is a systemic disease, which means its attack can charge on to other organs and parts of the body, including the eyes, lungs, and heart. Once again, and I can't stress this often enough, if you suspect that you may have arthritis, it is important to have it diagnosed by a medical professional.

The symptoms of arthritis

Arthritis cannot be diagnosed from just a few symptoms or a one-time occurrence of pain or inflammation. There are many factors that need to be considered when diagnosing arthritis:

- How long the pain lasts.
- How long you have had the symptoms and whether you have a history of them.
- What joints are affected. Any joint can be affected, but the joints that carry the most body weight, including the feet, knees, hips, and the fingers, are the most common.
- How severe the pain is.
- Whether medication has helped to alleviate any symptoms in the past.
- If you have the ability to bend and straighten the joint for normal activities.
- If there are other symptoms, such as numbness, stiffness, fever, or vomiting.

    Symptoms of arthritis also include:

- Tenderness.
- A grating feeling when you move the joint.

Unofficially...
Elephants never forget...pain. According to Dr. Harold Clark, an expert on arthritis in elephants, the great beasts suffer from morning stiffness, especially on cold mornings. One elephant even tested positive for the rheumatoid factor.

Bright Idea
If you suspect that you have arthritis, begin to keep a diary of all of your symptoms and what you were doing when they worsened. In addition, list the medications you are taking, how much and how often. This journal will be helpful when you consult your physician.

- Enlargement of the joint.

- Pain during motion.

- Fatigue.

- Low-grade fever.

- Malaise.

- Excessive weight loss or anorexia.

- Stiffness that may start throughout the body or on one part of your joint, such as the finger, and then gradually spread.

As we mentioned, arthritis means inflammation of the joint. Joint inflammation can include one or more of these symptoms: swelling, stiffness, tenderness, redness or warmth.

The inflammation of your joints is not necessarily something negative. It is your body's response to an infection or injury. It is the protection that your body needs to recuperate and heal. Your body responds to an infection or injury, also called a trigger, by sending fibroblasts, tissue-building cells, to the area. At the same time, chemical messengers, called cytokines and prostaglandins, control the healing process and enhance the cell growth. The entire process runs like a well-oiled machine. Well, almost.

Once the healing process is over, the inflammation should begin to subside, but this is not always the case. In some forms of arthritis, such as rheumatoid arthritis, once the immune system is done battling the infection or injury, it continues its drive to destroy, but since there are no foreign or damaged cells to fight, it begins to damage the normal tissues and cartilage of the joint.

This misdirection action is the hallmark of an autoimmune disorder—a disorder in which the body engages in battle with its own healthy tissue. Examples of autoimmune disorders within the arthritis family include rheumatoid arthritis, Graves disease, ankylosing spondylitis, and systemic lupus erythematosus.

The causes of arthritis

A faulty immune system is just one cause of arthritis. Unfortunately, scientists have not found the cause of all the 100 different types of arthritis. However, they have pinpointed several causes, including:

- Genetic predisposition: Genes are pockets of information that determine your physical characteristics, such as your gender, eye color, and height. Genes also carry health information. If you have a genetic predisposition to a disease, it means that you have a gene, or genetic marker, that makes you susceptible to this condition.

  For example, ankylosing spondylitis has been linked to the genetic marker HLA-B27 and rheumatoid arthritis has been linked to the genetic marker HLA-DR4. This means that if you have either of these genetic markers, you may have a genetically programmed susceptibility to developing that particular condition, if the right environmental conditions are met.

- Tumor necrosis factor: Scientists have also uncovered another possible cause of rheumatoid arthritis, the tumor necrosis factor, or TNF. TNF is a protein and chemical messenger, and is an important part of the body's normal means of fighting infection and injury. During chronic illnesses, the body may overproduce TNF to harmful levels. In turn, these high levels can exacerbate the symptoms of a chronic illness, such as rheumatoid arthritis.

66

I look okay on the outside, but people want to know why I am so slow or tired, or poop out fast. People who don't have arthritis or pain can't seem to understand what it's like to have fibromyalgia. My doctors would even tell me it was stress; it was typical to tell a woman she had stress.
—Joan, 48.

99

Unofficially...
A study by the National Institute of Arthritis and Musculoskeletal and Skin Diseases (NIAMSD) combined modern genetic research and century-old tribal records to pinpoint a gene that's possibly responsible for scleroderma, a connective tissue disease that affects Oklahoma Choctaw Native Americans. The disease affects all ethnic groups, but it's particularly prevalent among the Choctaw.

- Age: It has been mentioned before that age is not totally eliminated as a cause of arthritis. The risks for developing osteoarthritis simply increase because you are aging. The older you are, the more wear and tear your joints have been subjected to. This weakening of bones brought on by age and use make them more prone to breakdown, which can lead to arthritis.

- Long-term or ongoing abuse of a particular joint: Repetitive activities, like bowling, performed on a regular basis over the course of many years may make you prone to developing arthritis in that stressed joint.

- Viral, bacterial, or fungal infection: Rheumatoid arthritis, for example, is thought to be triggered by a virus in genetically prone individuals. Lyme disease, which can present arthritic symptoms, is a bacterial infection that is acquired through the bite of an infected deer tick. Transient arthritis is a form of arthritis that is caused by a viral infection such as the mumps, German measles, hepatitis B or parvovirus.

  Infectious arthritis is not usually a long-term, or chronic, illness. If it is treated promptly, it is one of the few curable forms of arthritis. Without proper treatment, however, infectious arthritis can damage the joints involved, and can spread to other parts of the body.

- Infecting organisms (otherwise known as reactive arthritis): Sometimes arthritis can start after an infection such as a sexually transmitted disease. It usually only involves one or two large joints. Anyone can develop reactive arthritis, but people who are most prone to this form include those who have medical illnesses such as diabetes or cancer, use intravenous recreational drugs, are engaging in unprotected sexual contact, or those treated with medications that lower the body's immune response.

Who gets arthritis?

While many forms of arthritis occur in both men and women, some of the most common and damaging attack women more frequently. According to the Arthritis Foundation, at least 26 million women of all ages are affected by some type of arthritis. This accounts for nearly two-thirds of all Americans living with the disease. Although the reasons are unclear, theories point to womens' weaker cartilage and tendons, and a possible link to the female sex hormone, estrogen, but this has yet to be proven. Here are some additional statistics on women and arthritis from the Arthritis Foundation:

- Osteoarthritis (OA) affects 15.3 million women (representing 74 percent of all cases).

- Rheumatoid arthritis (RA) affects 1.5 million women (representing 71 percent of all cases).

- Systemic lupus erythematosus (SLE) affects 117,000 women (representing 90 percent of all cases).

- Fibromyalgia affects an estimated 3.7 million Americans, mostly women.

- Juvenile rheumatoid arthritis (JRA) affects up to 50,000 children (with girls representing 86 percent of all cases).

Genes, ethnicity, and arthritis

Whether or not you develop arthritis may also depend on your ethnic background. For example, nearly four million African-Americans are affected

> **"**
> For the last three months my fatigue has been so severe that I cannot drive out of town, so I have to hire a driver or ask a friend to take me into the city as well. The expense of a chronic illness beyond what insurance covers is astronomical when you consider that it is neverending.
> —Michelle, 39
> **"**

Unofficially...
According to the Arthritis Foundation, osteo- and rheumatoid arthritis are the leading causes of work limitation among women. Earnings lost annually by women with arthritic symptoms are estimated at $8.9 billion, $3.2 billion of it due solely to arthritis. Individuals with advanced rheumatoid arthritis lose, on average, about 50 percent of the income they'd have earned had they not had arthritis.

by arthritis. It has been reported that African-American men are twice as likely as Caucasian men to have gout, a form of arthritis caused by uric crystals in the joints. Additionally, a much higher incidence rate of lupus occurs among African-Americans than Caucasians, with African-American women being three times more likely to be affected than Caucasian women.

Location, location, location...

Where you live may not be a risk factor of most types of arthritis, but it is a significant factor in Lyme disease, a bacterial form of arthritis. Lyme disease is a bacterial disease acquired through a tick bite. It is more commonly seen in New England states, such as Connecticut, Massachusetts, New Jersey, New York, and Rhode Island. The majority of the cases in those states are reported during the late spring and late summer, so visitors to those areas during that time are also at an increased risk.

How arthritis affects you

It is common thinking that people with arthritis are only hurting physically. Of course, there is the physical pain of the disease, but arthritis can also affect you emotionally, financially, and socially.

- Daily living: Arthritis can affect all aspects of your daily life, making it hard to perform even simple tasks. With arthritis, you may find it difficult to open bottles or cans, turn a doorknob, walk up a flight of stairs, or participate in myriad other everyday activities.

- Depression: Studies have shown that patients who live with chronic illness, such as arthritis, suffer from depression more than those who do not. Studies have also shown that this depression can exacerbate their medical conditions. For example, rheumatoid arthritis patients who have had even a single past episode of depression are at a greater risk for reporting pain, fatigue, and feeling disabled by their disease at a later date.

- Lowered self-esteem: According to the Arthritis Foundation study of 500 rheumatoid arthritis patients, 81 percent were frustrated by the feeling of no longer being in control; 32 percent reported they cannot get dressed when their rheumatoid arthritis is at its worst. Some arthritis patients must depend on others to help them with their daily needs. This may lead to a lowered self-esteem and a lack of self-worth. In addition, arthritis patients worry about their appearance and reactions of others to the physical symptoms of the disease, such as gnarled fingers and swollen joints.

- Side effects: Medications to help fight the pain and inflammation of arthritis are not without side effects. Sometimes, these side effects can cause additional problems. For example, many arthritis patients have gastrointestinal problems and ulcers resulting from medications that have irritated stomach lining. Other medications can cause rashes, hair loss, dry mouth, fatigue, and more.

- Financially: Arthritis can affect you financially, as well. Chronic pain and illness force many sufferers to quit their jobs, change careers, or retire early. This financial burden can also be exacerbated by mounting doctor bills, money for pain medication, or other medical necessities.

> 66
> I suddenly felt old when I found out I had arthritis (I got over it, but it was really not a happy time for awhile there). When you're still young and accustomed to a very independent life, it's hard to accept that you need a cane to get around, or that you can't wash your hair because you can't raise your arms that high in the shower.
> —Nancy, 46
> 99

Treatments

Treatment for the symptoms of arthritis depends on the type of arthritis that you have and the severity of your symptoms. Over the last half-century, scientists have made tremendous strides in the diagnosis and treatment of many forms of arthritis: For example:

- Gout was once a common, untreatable disease that debilitated those afflicted with this painful condition. Today gout is understood as a defect in body chemistry and can be almost completely controlled with medication and dietary changes.

- Lyme disease, now known as a trigger for rheumatoid arthritis, was a mysterious illness just 20 years ago. Once it was identified as a tick-borne illness, researchers have studied it and educated the public about prevention and treatment. In 1998, a vaccine was approved for use by anyone over 15 year of age to help prevent this condition, and if diagnosed early, it can be effectively treated with antibiotics.

- In the past, the treatment for arthritis often included rest and avoiding exercise. While rest is a vital part of any treatment plan, keeping bones and joints still for an extended period of time is now considered detrimental. Lack of physical activity results in muscular atrophy, or weakness, and stiffness in the joints. This causes reduced mobility, above and beyond what was initially caused by the arthritis. The Surgeon General's Report on Physical Activity and Health has even stated that osteoarthritis benefits from regular physical activity to maintain normal muscle strength, joint structure and joint function. Current medical treatment includes a regimen of physical activity.

■ Years ago, there was a limited selection of medications to help ease the pain and other symptoms of arthritis. Today, pharmaceutical advances have helped provide new methods to relieve the symptoms of arthritis. These medications include nonsteroidal, anti-inflammatory drugs (NSAIDs) that slow down the body's production of prostaglandins, substances that play a role in inflammation. They also carry some analgesic, or pain killing, properties as well. Another powerful class of medications are disease-modifying anti-rheumatic drugs (DMARDs), which work to slow or stop the basic progress of the disease. Conventional treatment includes a one-two combination punch of NSAIDs and DMARDs.

■ These medications have brought much needed relief to arthritis sufferers, but they have also brought intense side effects, especially an increased incidence of ulcers and other gastrointestinal problems. Scientists answered the need for a safer medication and, in just the past two years, have created medications that promise fewer gastrointestinal side effects than NSAIDs and aspirin. The first inhibitor, Celebrex, was introduced on the market early in 1999. Another medication, brand name Arava, is the first DMARD approved especially for rheumatoid arthritis treatment in more than 10 years. The drug blocks the overproduction of immune cells that are responsible for most of the inflammation. Enbrel is the first medication approved by the FDA to fight the tumor necrosis factor (TNF) of rheumatoid arthritis and was also introduced at the beginning of 1999. Enbrel eliminates, or "soaks up," excess TNF

Unofficially... An estimated 22.8 million adult women self-reported arthritis between 1989 to 1991. By the year 2020, an estimated 36 million adult women will be affected by arthritis.

> **"**
> I had back pain that severely impacted other areas of my body. I was diagnosed with mysterious cases of shoulder bursitis, plantar fascitis, carpal tunnel and tennis elbow...heck, I never even played tennis! I have always been sedentary, so I knew an underlying disease had to be causing all these problems. Believe it or not, I was thankful when I was finally diagnosed with psoriatic arthritis.
> —Michelle, 39
> **"**

before it can damage joints. Another potential TNF inhibitor, Remicade, is currently under review.

- Experts agree, however, that the greatest advance in the last few decades has been the advent of total joint replacement: the replacement of a diseased joint with an artificial prosthesis. Artificial joint replacement surgery is most commonly performed on hips and knees, but can also be performed on fingers, wrists, ankles, elbows, and shoulders. Artificial joint replacement is very successful surgery that has given new life to arthritis sufferers.

All of these advances in arthritis diagnosis and treatment have been received as "miraculous," especially by long-term sufferers of the disease. Nonetheless, more attention to the disease, its possible causes and its treatments is necessary, as it is predicted that more than 20 percent of the population will be diagnosed with arthritis in the next 25 years.

"It is projected that 60 million Americans, or 20 percent of the population, will have arthritis by the year 2020," cautions Dr. Sara Kramer, Chair of the Arthritis Foundation's New York chapter Government Affairs Committee and a rheumatologist affiliated with the New York University Medical Center. Because of this statistic and the crippling affect that arthritis can have on lives, a national health project from the Centers for Disease Control, called the National Arthritis Action Plan, has been put into action. This plan will hopefully help to reduce the financial and emotional burden of arthritis on Americans.

Just the facts

- Becoming familiar with your body will help you to stay healthy.

- Arthritis is not a condition you get when you get older. Arthritis can strike at any age, male or female.

- Modern science has seen many advancements in the treatment of arthritis symptoms.

- Arthritis is not just a condition of the body; it affects the mind as well.

- In severe cases, arthritis can be fatal.

GET THE SCOOP ON...
Finding a doctor ▪ What happens during
an exam ▪ Your guide to tests ▪ What the
results mean

Making a Diagnosis: Do You Have Arthritis?

Chapter 2

One of the most important factors in successfully treating and managing arthritis pain is to have it diagnosed as soon as possible to slow down the progression of the condition and reduce further damage to your joints. A simple case of aches and pains might not seem serious enough to motivate you to see a doctor, but if the pain persists, reoccurs, is accompanied by swelling or numbness, or is severe enough to interfere with your normal everyday activities, you really should seek medical attention.

Pain is your body's way of signaling you that there is something wrong, and as such it should never be ignored. That way you can get an early start on finding an appropriate treatment.

Hopefully, when you enter that doctor's office and complete diagnostic tests you will get answers to your questions. However, it is important to realize that the first step to diagnosing your pain is making sure you get to your doctor. This might sound crazy, but even when some people are in pain, they avoid the doctor. This is bad judgment. Certain forms of chronic arthritis can be debilitating and, if not treated early and properly, the disease can progress and interfere with other organs of the body. In severe cases, some forms of arthritis can be fatal. Avoiding the doctor is a mistake. Finding out what is causing your pain and being put on the road to recovery is most important in taking care of you.

There are many methods of diagnosing your pain, from blood tests to specialized genetic testing that determines if you are genetically susceptible to getting a particular form of arthritis. Unfortunately, to some degree, joint pain and inflammation are still mysteries. When you enter the doctor's office, you may be very eager to obtain answers to your questions. In some cases, you may not get any answers—or at least not right away. For those who suffer from rheumatoid arthritis and fibromyalgia, this can be especially frustrating. It may take months of tests and doctors and specialists and more tests before it is determined exactly what is causing your pain. In the meantime, you have to cope, then live each day the best that you can and know that, underneath it all, your symptoms are real.

The examination

Start with your primary care physician. If you are not a member of an HMO and do not have a primary care physician, it is important to select a doctor with whom you are comfortable, who looks for the causes of your symptoms, and does not simply prescribe painkillers. A complete examination will determine whether or not you are suffering from arthritis and, if so, which of the 100 types of arthritis you may have. The doctor can then begin the correct combination of treatment to alleviate your symptoms.

Your physician will perform a complete examination that includes:

- A complete medical history.
- An interview to discuss your symptoms.
- A physical examination.
- Additional lab tests or x-rays, if necessary.

These are the same parts of an examination that you would complete when you go for your annual physical. First, it is important to complete a full assessment of your health to rule out other possible illnesses or diseases. Second, what your physician will look for in these tests are results that point to arthritis. Based on the results of this complete examination, you may be referred to a specialist such as a rheumatologist, orthopedic surgeon, physical therapist, occupational therapist, or any combination of these professionals.

Medical histories

Your medical history and the medical histories of your immediate family members may provide some insight as to any inherited medical conditions. If this is your first visit to this doctor, obtain a copy of your medical records from your previous doctors to bring with you. Make notations of your parents or siblings who have suffered from any chronic illnesses.

The interview

Doctors will ask many questions about your symptoms. It is important to be open and honest with your doctor about all of your symptoms. It is also important to be specific when answering questions. For example, if you tell a doctor that you have joint pain, let him know in which joints. The symptoms will differ depending on the condition. Telling the

Bright Idea
If you do not belong to a medical plan that requires you to use a particular doctor, ask friends and family for references. For a list of doctors in your area, visit the American Medical Association's web site at www. ama-assn.org. for names, addresses, phone numbers and background information on a physician near you.

doctor that you have pain in all of your joints when it is only a few may mean the difference between a initial diagnosis of possible rheumatoid arthritis, which affects all of the joints, or osteoarthritis, which only affects some.

Some questions may include:

- How long does the pain last?

Timesaver
Maintain a journal of your symptoms—rank them on a scale of 1 to 10—to take to appointments. It will help the doctor to recognize patterns, such as morning pain, or underlying symptoms, such as a recent bout of the flu, which may contribute to your condition. Include when and where symptoms start, what you were doing, and how long they last.

- How long have you had the symptoms? Have you had any of them before? A sudden onset of arthritis pain may be an indication of gout, which is characterized by abnormally elevated levels of uric acid in the blood that causes hard lumps of uric acid to settle in the joints. Or in a more extreme case, a sudden onset of hot, painful joints may signify septic arthritis, a form of arthritis that usually occurs as a result of an injury to the joint. This type of arthritis is a medical emergency. However, if the pain is gradual, but worsening, it may be a sign of osteoarthritis, a degenerative form of arthritis that slowly deteriorates the joint.

- Describe the pain. Is it sudden and severe or slow and mild? When is it worse, during the day or at night? Morning stiffness happens to be one symptom of rheumatoid arthritis.

- Does medication help to alleviate any symptoms? If so, what do you take, how much and how often? Taking strong doses of pain relief medications for an extended period of time may trigger additional complications. As a result, the doctor may want to modify the dosage of your medication and perform additional tests to see if the medication is working and if it is causing any internal damage.

- Can you bend and straighten the joint and can you use it for normal activities? If your activities have been limited from the pain, explain what activities you are involved in.

- Are there any other symptoms, such as numbness, stiffness, fever, or vomiting?

- Have you had a recent injury to the area, or a disease, such as the flu, hepatitis, measles, or rheumatic fever? It is now known that certain viruses or infections can trigger arthritis, or mimic its symptoms. Remembering what you experienced before these symptoms began can help your diagnosis.

The physical examination
The doctor will conduct a physical examination. Most important, the doctor is looking for tenderness, limited range of motion or effusion—fluid collection around a joint. For example, if you are complaining of pain in your hands and wrists, the doctor may apply pressure on both wrists, or on a nearby tendon, at the same time and ask you to compare the pain. The doctor may also move the area to see if it triggers pain or if there is a limited range of motion. The doctor will look for any muscle spasms and joint deformities. When examining a child for possible juvenile arthritis, the physician may look for rashes, nodules or eye problems that may suggest the presence of juvenile arthritis.

Again, it is important to note that findings from a physical examination may not lead to an immediate diagnosis. For example, tenderness around the elbow joint may signify bursitis. However, when further evaluation is completed, it may be determined that you have rheumatoid arthritis, not bursitis.

Let's run some tests

Once the interview and physical examination are complete, the doctor will determine if additional testing is necessary. In many cases, it may not be possible or necessary to make an early diagnosis. The doctor may choose to wait an additional period of time and, in the meantime, treat the current symptoms. If any additional symptoms arise, the pain becomes severe, the symptoms have not diminished, or there is accompanying fever or weight loss, the doctor may order additional testing.

A physical examination of your joints and muscles can help the doctor make a diagnosis, but sometimes it just isn't enough. Blood and urine tests, x-rays, and biopsies (samples of skin or muscle tissue examined under a microscope) can provide clues to what is happening inside your body.

The most common tests that the doctor may prescribe include:

- Blood tests.
- Joint-fluid tests.
- X-rays.
- Urine tests.

Again, it is important to remember that the results of these tests may not provide all the answers you need. You may have to repeat tests, undergo new tests, or wait to see if the results change after time. This is all normal procedure and part of the diagnostic process for arthritis. If you have any questions regarding any test, however, make sure you ask first.

Blood will tell

By testing your blood, your doctor can turn up valuable clues as to precisely what type of arthritis is causing your aches and pains. These tests are of two general types: a complete blood workup, and more specialized tests designed to zero in on the source of your pain.

Complete blood test: A complete blood test is a simple method of evaluating red blood cells, white blood cells, and platelets, and is probably one of the most frequently performed lab tests. The main function of red blood cells is to transport oxygen, which is carried by the hemoglobin. The hematocrit (HCT) and hemoglobin (Hgb) tests measure the number and the quality of your red blood cells. If your red blood cell count is low, you might be experiencing chronic inflammation that results in pain, redness, swelling, and warmth of your joints.

The most important function of the white blood cells is to destroy bacteria, fungi and viruses that invade the body. The white blood cell count test (WBC) measures the amount of white blood cells that fight infection. If the number of white blood cells is too high or too low, an infection may be invading your body and causing your symptoms, such as lupus or rheumatoid arthritis.

Platelets are the sticky cells that help blood to clot. If your platelets are too low, your blood loses its ability to clot, which can cause excessive bleeding. This is important when your body is healing itself from injuries or illnesses. Low platelets are also associated with an increased risk of rheumatoid arthritis.

Powerful medications can also cause changes in your white and red blood cell count, so, once again, inform your physician of any medications you are currently taking.

Timesaver
Bring a list of questions you may have to your appointments. You may get nervous or anxious while listening to the doctor and forget what questions you have. A list will help you to remember and calm your fears that all of your concerns have been answered.

Specialized blood tests: There are also specialized blood tests that can help to diagnose arthritis symptoms:

- Erythrocyte sedimentation rate (ESR) test: Also called the "sed rate" test, it monitors how fast red blood cells cling together, fall, and settle to the bottom of a glass tube. The higher the sed rate, the greater the amount of inflammation you will have. This test helps to diagnose rheumatoid arthritis, lupus, scleroderma, systemic lupus erythematosus, Grave's disease, and other inflammatory diseases.

- Uric acid test: This measures the amount of uric acid in the blood and is used to diagnose gout, a condition that occurs when excess uric acid crystallizes and forms deposits in the joints and other tissues, causing inflammation and severe pain.

- Lyme serology blood test: Used to help diagnose Lyme disease. This blood test measures the presence of antibodies, which are produced by the body in response to the spirochete organism that enters the body via the tick's saliva. Unfortunately, in the early weeks of the infection, this blood test can be negative and fail to diagnose Lyme disease.

- Rheumatoid factor test: This test is ordered when there is a suspicion of rheumatoid arthritis. A rheumatoid factor is an abnormal antibody that is usually present in people with rheumatoid arthritis. The rheumatoid factor test is usually positive in people with rheumatoid arthritis. However, if you are tested for the RF factor, a positive test result does not mean that you will develop rheumatoid arthritis. Also,

25 percent or more patients with RA never have a positive RF. Therefore, the diagnosis should never be based solely on the results of RF testing. A positive test result may also indicate other autoimmune diseases, such as Sjogren's Syndrome, scleroderma, lupus, and dermatomyositis.

■ C-Reactive protein test: This checks for acute inflammation in conditions such as rheumatoid arthritis and lupus. C-reactive protein is produced by the liver during periods of inflammation.

Additional diagnostic tests

In addition to blood tests, your doctor may order several other specialized tests to pinpoint his or her diagnosis. A list of the more frequently used tests for arthritis includes:

Joint fluid test: Otherwise known as an arthrocentesis, a joint fluid test removes a small amount of synovial fluid, the fluid that lubricates the joint and helps it to bend. Joint fluid is normally clear and stringy, but when there is an infection, inflammation or trauma to the joint, the fluid will change in appearance. Most commonly, an arthrocentesis tests for the presence of white blood cells , protein, uric acid crystals, or bacteria and can help to diagnose gout and rheumatoid arthritis.

An arthrocentesis is a relatively safe procedure that is commonly performed on the knee with a local anesthetic.

X-rays: X-rays are a valuable tool in diagnosing many medical conditions, but x-rays are not very helpful in diagnosing certain forms of arthritis since it may take years for the bone damage to show up. X-rays are helpful, however, in showing changes of the bone that may indicate arthritis. X-rays can also monitor the damage of arthritis once it has begun. They can detect osteophytes, or small bone growths, that may signify ankylosing spondylitis, a painful progressive rheumatic disease that mostly affects the spine.

Special x-rays, called myelograms, can help diagnose any distortions of the spinal cord, spinal nerve roots, and the surrounding space. Myelograms are done by injecting a dye into the spinal canal before the x-ray is taken. The x-ray can detect any bulging discs that are pressing on nerves. These special x-rays can also eliminate other reasons for back pain. Computerized tomography is an x-ray technique that has now eliminated the use of the dye.

Watch Out!
If you are scheduled for an MRI, notify your physician and technician immediately if you wear a pacemaker, metallic aneurysm clips, metallic prostheses, or any metal foreign objects. Since these items can alter the test's results you cannot have this test done.

Magnetic resonance imaging (MRI): One alternative to x-rays is magnetic resonance imaging, which uses magnetism, radiowaves, and a computer, not radiation, to produce images of the body structure. The procedure is painless and there are no known side effects. It is becoming the procedure of choice for diagnosing a number of conditions. MRIs have the ability to see soft tissue and has become an important diagnostic tool in imaging muscles and bones.

The patient is put into a tunnel that is open at both ends. Still, some patients may feel uncomfortable in small spaces or experience claustrophobia. Since you must remain motionless for this procedure, ask your doctor for relaxation techniques or a mild sedative if you are worried you will be claustrophobic. Also, keep in mind that there are now many places that use "open MRIs"—the procedue in such cases is far less claustrophobic than the earlier version.

MRI scanning is very effective in evaluating orthopedic problems, such as degenerative arthritis of the spine, ankylosing spondylitis, and osteo-myelitis.

Anti-nuclear antibodies: Anti-nuclear antibodies, otherwise known as ANA titers, are measured to detect the presence of antibodies that are found in conjunction with a variety of autoimmune diseases, such as rheumatoid arthritis, scleroderma, and systemic lupus erythematosus. Certain medications, however, can cause a false positive on this test, so it is important to notify your physician if you are taking antibiotics, birth control pills, corticosteroids, tranquilizers or thiazide diuretics.

Testing for bone loss: Bone density tests are important to determine the extent of your bone loss. These tests are especially important for women once they reach menopause. The production of estrogen, a hormone that strengthens bone, begins to decline at menopause and women become at a higher risk for bone loss. This increases the risk of osteoporosis, otherwise known as "brittle bone disease," or thinning of bone tissue and the growth of small holes in the bone. Osteoporosis can cause pain in the lower back, frequent broken bones, and loss of body height.

If the results of a bone density test indicate low bone mass, your doctor may suggest treatment. Treatment may include calcium supplements, or estrogen replacement therapy. The World Health Organization does not recommend bone testing for everyone, but does recommend the testing if:

- You regularly use steroids, heparin, thyroxine, multiple anticonvulsants, or alcohol and are not on estrogen replacement therapy.

- You have rheumatoid arthritis, hyperthyroidism, Type I diabetes, chronic liver or kidney

Moneysaver
MRIs are still very costly, and may not be covered by all medical insurance plans. If you are scheduled to have an MRI done, call your insurance company and verify that you are covered so you do not get stuck with the bill. Also do not bring your wallet into the examining room, as the test can erase all the magnetic strips on your credit cards. Instead, have a family member hold on to your wallet.

disease, or a family history of osteoporosis, and are not on estrogen replacement therapy.

■ You experienced menopause before age 45 and aren't taking estrogen.

■ An x-ray suggests osteoporosis or low bone mass.

Dual-energy x-ray absorptiometry (DEXA or DXA) is one type of bone density test that measures bone loss in your spine and hips. It can detect even a one-percent bone loss. DEXA is a short procedure (usually 10 to 15 minutes) that consists of lying on a padded platform while a mechanical wand-like device scans your body. The amount of radiation from this procedure is only a fraction of what is used in a chest x-ray. Not all insurance carriers cover DEXA tests, so check with your carrier before having the test done.

Genetic testing: One of the most remarkable discoveries of this century is the fact that scientists have identified genes, or genetic markers, which cause some types of arthritis. For example, researchers have discovered that ankylosing spondylitis is usually present in people who have the genetic marker HLA-B27. White blood cells are then tested for the presence of the genetic marker HLA-B27. This test can also determine if you have the genetic factor for Reiter's syndrome.

Researchers have also discovered the "rheumatoid factor"—known in the scientific literature as RA factor HLA-DR4. This appears to be a genetic marker on the surface of the cells that indicates an inherited tendency toward developing rheumatoid arthritis. This rheumatoid factor is an abnormal substance that occurs in the blood of about 80 percent of adults with rheumatoid arthritis.

Moneysaver
Get copies of your previous x-rays, especially if they were done recently. This will save money, especially if you are required to pay a per–x-ray charge. Also, if your physician orders an entire-body x-ray, ask questions. Since most types of arthritis do not affect every bone, this is usually a waste of time and money.

Genetic screening can determine if you are a carrier of the gene that carries a particular disease. The testing is done through a simple blood sample or through a sample of cells obtained from inside the mouth.

By pinpointing these specific gene markers that carry or cause the disease, scientists can now research the process of eliminating the defective gene. Discovering these gene markers will also lead to additional treatments for the conditions.

Urine tests: A urinalysis can be evaluated within 24 hours to see if the urine contains red blood cells, protein or other abnormal substances. This may indicate kidney damage or medications that can cause loss of kidney function. Kidney damage is a symptom of some rheumatic diseases such as lupus.

Biopsies: Taking small samples of skin, muscle, or kidney tissue and examining it under a microscope can help to confirm various types of arthritis. For example, skin biopsies can diagnose lupus and psoriatic arthritis; muscle biopsies can help to detect polymyositis, a connective tissue disease. Skin and muscle biopsies are relatively painless and done under local anesthetic, but there will be a small scar. No hospitalization is needed. Less frequently used biopsies include synovial, lung, salivary gland, and blood vessel.

Creatinine test: In some rheumatic diseases, the damage from arthritis has already started. Damaged muscles will release enzymes into the blood that are picked up by muscle enzyme tests, such as the creatinine phosphokinase and aldolase tests. A serum creatinine test is used to determine the level of creatinine, a normal waste product of the muscles that is in the blood. High levels of creatinine may signify that the kidneys are not working properly to remove this waste product. This indicates a symptom of lupus or other connective tissue diseases.

Arthroscopy: Arthroscopy is a surgical procedure that examines the interior of a joint via a camera-like instrument that is inserted through small incisions made at the joint. The results of the arthroscopy are used to diagnose or treat joint abnormalities including:

- Torn cartilage in the knee or shoulder.

- Reconstruct the ligaments in the knee.

- Remove inflamed joint tissues, also known as a synovectomy. The tissue lining can then be biopsied and examined under a microscope to determine the cause of the inflammation.

- Release of carpal tunnel.

- Remove loose bone or cartilage in knee, shoulder elbow, ankle or wrist.

The surgery is minimally invasive and you will be given either a general, spinal, or local anesthetic. An arthroscope, a small tube that contains optical fibers and lenses, is inserted through tiny incisions in the skin and into the joint that is being examined. The tube projects pictures of the joint onto a television monitor for the surgeon to see.

Post-diagnostic testing

Once you are diagnosed with arthritis, there may be further testing at a later date to see how the symptoms are responding to treatment. Additional tests may also be necessary to make certain there are no complications from the arthritis, or to monitor the medication and watch for any side effects. Some of these tests include:

- Salicylate level tests: salicylate is the main ingredient in aspirin and some non-steroidal anti-inflammatory drugs. High levels of salicylate can cause ringing in the ears, fever, nausea, vomiting, rapid breathing, headache, and irritability. In severe cases it can cause convulsions and breathing failure.

- Muscle enzyme tests: creatinine phosphokinase and aldolase tests can detect muscle damage that may be caused by certain medications.

- Liver enzyme tests: measures the amount of liver damage caused by certain medications, including NSAIDs and aspirin.

Analyzing the results

No matter how long you have been experiencing your symptoms, you will be quite eager for the results once you have completed the tests. Knowing that you may have some answers can be a relief, but sometimes the answers may even leave you with more unanswered questions.

When the test comes back positive

A positive test result does not always mean that you will develop the disease. For example, in the early stages of rheumatoid arthritis, only one in five people test positive for rheumatoid factor, but 15 to 20 percent of those who have rheumatoid arthritis never test positive.

If you have been diagnosed with a form of arthritis, it is important to gain as much knowledge as you can about it. Ask your doctor questions, read books on the subject, or contact arthritis organizations for more information. Knowing as much as you can about the causes, symptoms, and treatments of your particular arthritis is an important step in coping

Bright Idea
Any time you are scheduled for medical tests, ask your doctor how to prepare for them. Do you need to fast or eliminate certain foods from your diet? Some tests require that you stop taking certain medications beforehand. Antibiotics, oral contraceptives, steroids, and tranquilizers can affect some test results.

Moneysaver
Don't run from doctor to doctor just because you do not like what the doctors are saying. Most insurance companies do not cover more than a second opinion, so this can be costly to you. If your second opinion agrees with your first, follow your doctor's advice and let some time go by. Other symptoms may arise that could provide a clearer picture.

with the condition and putting yourself on the road to recovery.

Tests can't tell it all

While lab tests have their utility, they all have limitations. For example, a test may come back with a false negative or a false positive. The point is that lab testing is only one of many tools in your doctor's repertoire, and should not be relied upon exclusively.

Other reasons why lab tests may not provide the answers you are looking for:

- Symptoms can overlap. "Mixed connective tissue disease" is actually a name of three diseases that have similar symptoms. These conditions (systemic lupus erythematosus, scleroderma, and polymyositis) can occur together.

- Symptoms may also evolve slowly. You may only have achy joints now, but additional symptoms may not show up for another year. However, it does not mean that you are not experiencing legitimate pain. It just may take some time to develop a diagnosis.

  For example, as discussed earlier, if blood tests are performed for Lyme disease too early (before the first three to four weeks after the bite from an infected tick) a person may get a false negative test result because his immune system may not have produced a large enough amount of antibodies to be detected. The test will be read as negative even though the person does indeed have Lyme disease. In this case, monitoring the symptoms is vital and another blood test should be done at a later time if the symptoms remain after a few weeks.

- You may be suffering from several health problems at once. For example, a low red blood cell count may signify the beginning of an arthritic condition, and it may also be an indication of low iron in your blood. This is often the case with older people who complain of joint pain. X-rays may show signs of osteoporosis, but the person may also have osteoarthritis as well.

Depending on the test results, the management of your condition may be just a few reassuring words, medication, or reassessment at a later date. The treatment will also depend on your age, what type of arthritis you may have, and other any medical conditions. Your doctor may refer you to a specialist for further evaluation, such as a:

Bright Idea
Bring somebody with you to the examination for emotional support.

- Rheumatologist: An internist or pediatrician who has had additional training in the diagnosis and treatment of arthritis or juvenile arthritis and related disorders of the joints, bones, and muscles.

- Physical therapist: strengthens muscles to support your joints and teaches you simpler ways of dressing, walking, climbing stairs, and bathing.

- Occupational therapist: helps you to both improve the range of motion in the affected joint and strengthen the muscles that support the joint. Provides you with helpful devices, such as canes, crutches, or splints that can temporarily rest a sore joint.

- Neurologist: Assesses nerve damage to the affected area. Can provide treatment to stimulate nerves.

Just the facts

- Undergoing many tests to diagnose your symptoms is a routine part of medical care.

- Ruling out some forms of arthritis is just as important as diagnosing exactly what type that you have.

- Do not undergo any testing without thoroughly understanding the test, the possible outcomes and the risks involved.

- Diagnosing your condition may not be a cut-and-dried situation. Additional tests, waiting for time to pass and visits to specialists may have to take place before you find out the reasons for your pain and other symptoms.

The Many Faces
of Arthritis

PART II

Chapter 3

GET THE SCOOP ON...
Whether you are at risk ▪ Minimizing your
odds ▪ How to lessen the hurt ▪ Surgery: a
successful option

Osteoarthritis

The old adage says "you can be sure of two things in your life: death and taxes." Add one more: You can be sure that you will get some form of osteoarthritis by the time you are 75 years old. Currently, over 80 percent of the population aged 65 and over has the disease.

But it's not just older people who get osteoarthritis. Even if your golden years are still a lifetime away, osteoarthritis can strike. After all, it is not just a disease of the aging, but a degenerative disease of the joints that can affect those as young as 40 years old. If you have ever woken up feeling a little stiff, injured a joint in your body, carry a little extra weight, or are a woman, there's a good chance the process has already begun and you might not even realize it. Osteoarthritis affects 16 million people in the United States, but according to research, 40 million people would show evidence of the disease if they had an x-ray taken.

Bone on bone pain

In a healthy joint, two cartilage-covered bones meet, and the rubbery cartilage enables the joint to move freely. Over time, the cartilage begins to break down from normal, everyday wear and tear. In osteo-arthritis, the cartilage breaks down prematurely and exposes bone to rub against bone.

To visualize this process, take two rocks and rub them together. Without any cushion between the rocks, they rub against each other, creating possible hazards such as chipping and cracking. Bones are even more fragile than rocks and are more suscepti-ble to injury.

Now if you hit the rocks together hard enough, it might even cause a spark. For those who suffer from the pain of osteoarthritis, this spark is analo-gous to the pain they experience on a daily basis, making simple tasks such as opening a can or walk-ing the dog difficult.

This doesn't mean, however, that this chronic condition has to impact your entire lifestyle. You can minimize your risks at any age, or decrease any already existing discomfort. In this chapter, we'll show you how to determine if you are at risk for osteoarthritis and the proper treatment to make sure this chronic condition doesn't affect your work and family, or tarnish your golden years.

The risk factors of osteoarthritis

Osteoarthritis is the most common and oldest known form of arthritis, but the exact cause is not yet known. There are factors, however, that can increase your risk of developing osteoarthritis in the future, including:

- **Age:** Although osteoarthritis is not an inevitable part of aging, age is an important risk factor,

Unofficially...
Osteoarthritis accounts for more than seven million visits to doctors each year due to pain and decreased mobility. Osteoarthritis also accounts for 36 million lost workdays.

and your risk of developing osteoarthritis increases after age 45. Think of all the bending, walking, stretching, running, and jumping you have done in your lifetime. Every day, your joints support all of your activities from carrying groceries up the stairs to your aerobics class. When you participate in sports or exercise classes, your joints are also bearing the impact of your workout. Your joints simply break down over time.

■ **Injury to the joint:** Anyone who has suffered a repetitive motion injury or trauma to any joint is also at a greater risk for osteoarthritis. For example, assembly line workers or baseball pitchers who perform the same daily repetitive motion for hours on end might experience a cartilage breakdown in their elbows, wrists, or shoulders.

Although osteoarthritis affects mostly your spine, hips, knees, and feet—or the joints of your body that bear the majority of your weight—other joints can be affected as well, including your elbows, shoulders, and fingers.

■ **Gender:** Unfortunately, just being a woman also puts you into the risk-factor category. Out of the 16 million people afflicted with osteoarthritis, almost 12 million are women. Although the reasons are unclear, theories point to weaker cartilage and tendons in the joints as compared to men, and a possible link to estrogen, but results of studies on this have not been consistent.

■ **Weight:** If you are carrying excess weight, your bones and joints, especially your knees, hips, and ankles, must work harder to support those extra pounds. If you already have osteoarthritis, the excess weight can make your symptoms worse. Avoiding excess weight gain or losing excess weight can help you to lower your risk of developing osteoarthritis and can also help to ease any symptoms that you already have.

- **Activity level:** After what we have already discussed, you might think that it makes sense to stay off your joints to decrease your risk of osteoarthritis. This may sound like heaven for couch potatoes, but unfortunately, lack of activity can actually increase your risk. After all, when you are sedentary, your joints stiffen and your muscles weaken. Just to give you an idea of this: Remember how stiff you feel when you get up after sitting in a movie theater for a long period of time? Being sedentary leaves you prone to injury and to developing osteoarthritis. Exercise is one of the first recommended forms of preventing and treating osteoarthritis.

- **Genetic inheritance:** Recent findings have shown there may be a genetic predisposition to osteoarthritis, so if your parents have osteoarthritis, there is a chance that you might have it too. In one study, researchers isolated the same defective gene in a family where three members suffered from osteoarthritis. In another study, researchers examined x-rays of more than 600 pairs of female twins, both fraternal and identical, over the age of 40. Three of the four indicators showed that genetic influences are responsible for at least 50 percent of hip osteoarthritis.

This gene may contribute to a deficient cartilage or an improper structure of the joint. The gene will already predetermine that the normal operation of your joint will be altered and the cartilage will break down. If you have family members who have osteoarthritis, it is even more important for you to reduce your risks.

What are the symptoms?

The symptoms of osteoarthritis vary from person to person. One individual may have some general stiffness each morning that never progresses into much more. Another person might have severe, crippling pain all day long. If you have osteoarthritis, you can expect to experience one or more of the following symptoms:

- **Pain:** This can range from mild discomfort to a stabbing pain in the joints. In most cases, the pain subsides when the joint isn't being used. The weight-bearing joints (your hips, knees, and feet) are the most susceptible to osteoarthritis, but the pain can also be experienced in your neck, hands, and spine.

- **Stiffness:** It's a Catch-22: If you rest, the pain may subside; if you rest, the joints may stiffen up. Most likely you will feel stiff after you have been sitting for awhile, or after you wake up in the morning, but the stiffness should start to subside a few minutes after you begin to move around. Back and neck stiffness can also be caused by slow deterioration of the discs between the bones along your spine.

- **Inflammation:** Inflammation is a common symptom in rheumatoid arthritis, but is not as common in osteoarthritis. However, when a joint is overused, it can become warm, red, and inflamed.

Unofficially... Can switching from high heels to flats decrease your chances of developing osteoarthritis? Maybe. One England-based study claims that women who walk in high-heeled shoes strain the area between the kneecap and the thighbone, especially in the inner side of the knee joint. This joint strain may contribute to osteoarthritis, but further evaluation is needed.

- **Limited range of motion:** You might find it difficult to perform daily tasks, such as grasping door handles, turning a page, or walking up the stairs. The joint damage prevents the joint from flexing and bending normally.

- **Gnarled fingers:** When the fingers are affected, bony knobs can form and enlarge your finger joints, causing your fingers to look gnarled. These knobs are also referred to as Heberden's nodes. Abnormal swelling of knuckles, called Bouchard's nodes, is also a symptom of osteoarthritis. In most cases, these nodes affect more women than men and can take from weeks to years to appear.

Diagnosing the pain

When you visit your physician, you can expect:

- A physical evaluation.

- To detail your medical history.

- To have x-rays made of the affected joints.

- To undergo blood tests to eliminate the possibility of other forms of arthritis.

  These diagnostic tests are tools to help your physician determine if you have osteoarthritis. In some cases, you may also undergo an MRI. Chapter Two goes into these tests in greater detail.

Minimizing the risks

Exercise, eating right, and maintaining a healthy weight are important for a healthy body, and your joints benefit greatly from this as well. Excess pounds place undue stress on joints and can lead to a more rapid deterioration of the cartilage. A healthy nutritional plan can provide your body with all the nutrients it needs for strong bones and muscles and help you to eliminate excess weight.

Exercise and pain relief

Imagine carrying a very heavy bag of groceries. You might struggle and ache to put the bag down. When you do, you feel relieved, and your joints have a little less pressure to carry around. Then imagine losing the excess 10 or 20 pounds you're lugging around. Your joints will feel even better and you may slow down any already existing degeneration.

A Surgeon General's Report on Physical Activity and Health found that regular physical activity is necessary for maintaining normal muscle strength, joint structure, and joint function. Exercise was also not associated with joint damage or development of osteoarthritis. It has been found to be beneficial for many people with arthritis. This was true even for older adults with arthritis.

Exercise helps your body by doing the following:

- Strengthening the muscles that surround the joint, which can help absorb shock and improve its stability.

- Increasing the flexibility of the joint, which may lessen the pain.

- Improving posture, an important benefit to allow the joint to move properly. Improper posture can lead to muscle spasms and aches in the joints.

- Allowing the joint to soak up "good" fluid. When a cartilage moves inside a joint, it squeezes the water out of the joint. The "dry" cartilage soaks up new fluid that contains healthy nutrients and oxygen. The more a joint

Watch Out!
Consult your doctor before you begin any exercise program. You might need a physical therapist or physician to create an exercise program that is individualized to take into account any special needs due to your arthritis. Exercising without guidance can cause new or further injuries.

moves, the more fluid it soaks up and the more the joint is lubricated.

Studies on exercise and osteoarthritis prove the theory that you can cut your risk of developing osteoarthritis by more than half just by exercising. One study done over an 18-month period on those 60 and older with osteoarthritis of the knee who participated in regular exercise said the participants had consistent improvement.

Exercise also helps you lose weight by burning extra calories. Research shows that men who carry as little as 20 extra pounds in early adulthood nearly double their chances of developing painful knee and hip osteoarthritis. It's obvious that by exercising, you are receiving a multitude of healthy benefits for your entire body—and especially your joints.

Be careful, though. High-impact activities, such as basketball or jogging, can place too much stress on your joints and might cause more harm than good. For example, when you jump, your joints are absorbing the impact of almost 10 times your body weight. If you weigh 150 pounds, this means that your hips, knees, and ankles are carrying 1,500 pounds when you jump. Then add in any twisting motions and your joints are really taking a beating. Instead, low-impact or non-impact activities, such as walking or swimming, are less stressful on the joints.

Eating for relief

As a kid, you were probably told thousands of times to "eat right and you will grow up to be big and strong." If you did not pay attention, don't worry. There is always time to make improvements, although you cannot reverse any damage to your bones and joints that has already begun. Eating right means eating a variety of foods to get the vitamins, minerals, and protein your body needs to stay healthy.

You were also probably told to drink your milk, that it's good for your bones. Seems that Mom was right. Milk contains calcium and Vitamin D, which help promote bone growth and strength. Vitamin D isn't actually a vitamin, but a hormone processed in the liver and kidneys from chemicals activated by sunlight. Some studies have shown that Vitamin D appears to protect against the advancement of osteoarthritis. In addition to milk, you can also find Vitamin D in fish, eggs, some fortified cereals, and multivitamin supplements. Exposure to sunlight also helps synthesize it in your body.

As explained in Chapter One, calcium helps to build and maintain strong bones by slowing the amount of bone loss as you age. You can find calcium in dairy products, such as milk, cheese, and yogurt, and in dark green leafy vegetables, such as broccoli or bok choy.

The Recommended Daily Allowance of calcium is 800 milligrams for adults age 25 and older, but it is believed that you need more to prevent the bone loss that comes from aging.

Watch your weight to reduce the aches

Your body mass index (BMI) is an estimate of your body mass, including fat. It has been shown that a high BMI (over 25) can contribute to osteoarthritis. This number can also tell you how dangerous fat is for you.

The Mayo Clinic of Rochester, Minnesota provides a relatively simple formula for determining your BMI, although it should be done by a medical professional who can perform a thorough exam and explain the results to you. (The Mayo Clinic also

Moneysaver
Forget those fad diets. Do not waste money on books that focus on one "miracle" diet food. There is no such thing. For free information on healthy eating, check out the web site of the American Dietetic Association at http://www.eatright.org. The ADA also offers a Consumer Nutrition Hot Line at (800) 366-1655.

offers an informative chart on BMI on their web site: http://www.mayo.ivi.com)

1. Multiply your weight in pounds by 0.45. For example, if you weigh 150: $150 \times 0.45 = 68$

2. Multiply your height in inches by 0.025. For example, if you're 5'6" (66 inches): $66 \times 0.025 = 1.65$

3. Square the answer from step 2 ($1.65 \times 1.65 = 2.72$)

4. Divide the answer from step 1 by the answer from step 3 ($68 \div 2.72 = 25$)

Your BMI should fall within the healthy range of 19 to 25. If you are at the upper end of this range or score more than 25, consider losing enough weight to lower your BMI at least one or two numbers. A BMI of more than 27 is considered overweight and at a higher risk for osteoarthritis.

Estrogen and osteoarthritis

Estrogen is a female hormone that helps make your bones strong. As you age, you steadily lose the amount of estrogen in your body, which can lead to brittle bones. Estrogen replacement therapy helps to prevent such conditions. Researchers have studied estrogen as a means of protecting against osteoarthritis in elderly women. So far, the results have been positive, but more research is needed.

In addition, researchers found women currently receiving supplemental estrogen for 10 years or longer had a greater reduction in the risk of any hip osteoarthritis as compared to those who took it for less than 10 years. Past use of estrogen was not associated with a lower risk of hip osteoarthritis, but more research is needed.

Treatment strategies

No one treatment or combination of treatments can cure arthritis. But there are treatments to reduce pain and inflammation and help you to live a more productive life. Finding the right combination of treatments to manage your symptoms may take time, however, so be patient.

Rest and rejuvenate those joints

Years ago, rest was considered the cure for pain. Getting off your feet and elevating the painful area for a lengthy period of time was supposed to help alleviate the pain. Today, however, it has been discovered that while moderate rest is fine, prolonged inactivity will decrease muscle tone and overall health and fitness. Rest periods, incorporated with an exercise program, are essential to help control pain and inflammation.

When you are resting, alternate hot and cold packs on the affected area. Heat is used to soothe and relax the joint and the surrounding muscles. Cold packs numb the area, and decrease swelling and pain by constricting the blood vessels, thus reducing blood flow and fluid buildup. Alternate hot and cold packs for 20 minutes each, but do not continue applications longer than 20 minutes at a time. Your skin should be allowed to return to normal temperature between applications. Many people afflicted with arthritis often use a hot tub, heated pool, or hot shower to help loosen their stiff joints.

Support your joints and they'll support you

There are braces available that claim to create a normal or near-normal joint alignment while redistributing the weight on the joint. Braces may

Bright Idea
Give your child a head start on healthy bones. Pregnant and breast-feeding women should consume 1,200 milligrams of calcium daily.

Moneysaver
There are medical supply stores and catalogs that sell arthritis aids, such as door openers and walkers, to help make everyday living easier (see Chapter 14). If you can't afford to pay full price for these items, check the "for-sale" sections of your local newspaper, the bulletin boards at grocery stores, or garage sales.

alleviate some of the pain and enable you to better control the movement of your joint.

Dulling the pain

There is an ever-increasing number of drugs that can combat the inflammation and pain from arthritis. It is important for you to become knowledgeable about the most effective medications *and* their side effects. Here's a list of the more commonly used pain relievers:

- **Aspirin.** This is probably the first thing most people reach for to cope with arthritis pain. It is cheap and effective, but it can also irritate your gastrointestinal tract, which can lead to bleeding. If you take aspirin, take a brand that has an enteric coating. While an enteric coating means less stomach irritation because the pill does not release its contents until it reaches your intestines, it may take longer to obtain pain relief. In some cases, aspirin must be prescribed at very high doses; if so, your doctor will closely monitor you for side effects.

- **Acetaminophen.** If you cannot tolerate aspirin, the better choice for you may be acetaminophen, an aspirin-free pain reliever and fever reducer found in Tylenol and other brands. Acetaminophen is safe when used as directed, but side effects include severe anemia. Overdose can result in fatal liver failure. And when taken in conjunction with alcohol ingestion, liver damage can occur.

- **Nonsteroidal anti-inflammatory drugs (NSAIDs).** Generic versions include ibuprofen and naproxen; over-the-counter brands of NSAIDs include Advil, Nuprin, Motrin, and

Aleve. NSAIDs are considered to be less toxic than aspirin, but can still cause gastrointestinal bleeding and kidney problems in some patients. Inflammation is not a common symptom of osteoarthritis, unlike other forms of arthritis. Pain relief is the primary goal. NSAIDs work by slowing down the body's production of prostaglandins, substances that play a role in inflammation. They also carry some analgesic, or pain killing, properties as well. NSAIDs can be used if a patient does not respond to acetaminophen, but they must be carefully monitored for side effects, which include stomach trouble, gastric or duodenal ulceration, dizziness, skin rashes, and ringing in the ears. To prevent some of the gastrointestinal irritation, it is recommended that NSAIDs be taken with at least eight ounces of water. You are also advised not to lie down from 15 to 30 minutes after taking the drug.

- **Arthrotec.** If you are at high risk for gastrointestinal complications, there may be relief in sight. Arthrotec, the brand name for diclofenac sodium, received U.S. marketing clearance from the FDA for osteoarthritis patients who are at a high risk for ulcers and other complications caused by NSAIDs. Arthrotec consists of an enteric-coated core containing diclofenac sodium and misoprostol. There are side effects, however, including abdominal pain, diarrhea, and stomach upset. Women who are pregnant or plan to become pregnant should discuss the use of Arthrotec with their physicians.

- **Cox-2 Inhibitors.** Cox-2 inhibitors are a new class of painkillers that promise to cause fewer gastrointestinal side effects than NSAIDs and aspirin. Cox-2 is an enzyme that has been found to be the cause of the gastrointestinal distress associated with NSAIDs. Celebrex is the first Cox-2 inhibitor approved by the FDA for sale, but the FDA claims that research has not proven that Celebrex has fewer side effects than the other medications.

The FDA is also currently reviewing Vioxx, another Cox-2 inhibitor for treating osteo-arthritis. The makers of this drug tout its fewer gastrointestinal side effects than NSAIDs. Additional information on Vioxx should be available this year.

▪ **Disease-modifying anti-rheumatic drugs.** The heavy hitters in the medication team are a class commonly referred to as DMARDs: disease-modifying anti-rheumatic drugs. These drugs work to slow or stop the basic progress of the disease. You may have to take them for several weeks or months before you notice any signs of improvement. The side effects can be great, so these medications are reserved for severe and progressive diseases.

▪ **Topical pain relievers.** These are creams, sprays, or rubs that you apply on your skin over a sore muscle or joint to temporarily relieve the pain. Each pain reliever works differently, depending on its ingredients. For example, some contain salicylates, the pain relief substance found in aspirin. Others contain ingredients such as skin irritants, menthol, camphor, or capsaicin, the substance in chili peppers that makes them hot. Capsaicin creams block the ability of the nerve endings around the joint to send pain messages to the brain. Capsaicin appears to have no side effects, but some people experience burning or stinging after first applying the cream.

- **Corticosteroids.** Corticosteroids are synthetic versions of the hormone cortisone and include prednisone and dexamethasone. Cortisone is a steroid hormone that is produced in the liver, but can be made artificially and used to treat swelling. Corticosteroids are generally prescribed as short-term relief for an intense flare-up to immediately reduce pain and inflammation. Corticosteroids may also be used when patients do not find relief with other painkillers. Unfortunately, while the relief is quick and dramatic, there are serious side effects when corticosteroids are used over a long period of time. These side effects may include weight gain, high blood pressure, and thinning of the bones and skin. Therefore, the shots are not usually given more than a few times a year.

- **Synvisc and Hyalgan.** In 1998, the FDA granted approval for Synvisc and Hyalgan, known generically as sodium hyaluronate, to be marketed as pain relief medications for osteoarthritis of the knee. Sodium hyaluronate is a cushioning fluid normally found in the knees, but due to the cartilage degeneration, the joint is lacking this fluid. An injection of either chemical can prevent the irritation when the bones of the joint rub together. The treatment consists of three injections during a two-week period and is reserved for patients who do not respond well to other painkillers. Research shows that these substances reduce pain in the knee for about six months, but the injections are expensive. The

Watch Out!
The American Medical Association warns anyone who is allergic to aspirin or taking an anti-clotting medication to talk to their doctor before you use any rubs, creams or sprays that contain salicylates.

Unofficially...
The companies that developed hyaluronate, Italy's Fidia Corp. and New Jersey's Biomatrix, Inc., culled the substance from the combs of roosters and then modified it for humans.

three shots cost approximately $500. Make sure your insurance plan covers the cost beforehand.

The controversial supplements: glucosamine and chondroitin sulfate

No other treatment for osteoarthritis has received the consumer attention that these two products have. Within weeks of the publication of *The Arthritis Cure*, by Jason Theodosakis, M.D., of the University of Arizona College of Medicine, the book was on the *New York Times* best-seller list and the sales of the dietary supplements glucosamine and chondroitin skyrocketed. But while consumers who either have osteoarthritis or are at risk for developing the condition were quick to try the supplements, medical experts were not as quick to support the claims made in the book.

Glucosamine is a substance that is synthesized by the body and can play a role in repairing cartilage. It is believed that it may stimulate cartilage cells to grow and may inhibit the enzymes that break down this process. Chondroitin is another substance occurring naturally in cartilage, and Dr. Theodosakis claims that it can also stop the enzymes that break down the cartilage. He claims that combining these two substances boosts the actions of each.

However, according to the American Academy of Orthopaedic Surgeons, glucosamine and chondroitin sulfate may be generating statistically significant sales, but little evidence exists to show that these products relieve chronic joint pain. The American College of Rheumatology and the Arthritis Foundation also do not recommend these dietary supplements as a preventative measure for osteoarthritis. Both organizations have publicly stated that further studies are needed before any formal support of the products can be made. Interestingly, it is also noted on these products that "these statements have not been evaluated by the Food and Drug Administration. This product is not intended to diagnose treat or cure any disease."

Pinpricks for pain relief

Acupuncture is an ancient treatment that has been noted to cure hundreds of ailments for thousands of years in eastern civilization. It is now gaining popularity in conventional medicine as pain relief for osteoarthritis sufferers.

A study reported in 1997 by the University of Maryland says that acupuncture may play a useful role in the treatment of osteoarthritis of the knee. This treatment, in combination with conventional medical therapy, significantly improved pain and disability scores. However, additional studies are needed to determine the efficacy of acupuncture maintenance therapy, as well as the use of acupuncture in patients with early disease and milder symptoms.

Going the surgical route

Surgery might sound like a "when all else fails" option, but to many sufferers, it's the best one. The advances over the past 20 years in joint replacement surgery has been remarkable. Today, this surgery can dramatically improve the use of the affected limb and give independence to an otherwise dependent, activity-limited patient.

One type of surgery, arthroscopy, can be used to either diagnose or treat osteoarthritis. The surgery is performed by an orthopedic surgeon, a specialist in surgery on bones and joints. During arthroscopy, the doctor inserts a long viewing tube, called an arthroscope, into small incisions in the skin. The

Watch Out!
If you have been prescribed a painkilling medication, ask your doctor how the medication works and what its side effects are. Be sure to notify your physician and your pharmacist about any other drugs you are taking. Combining certain drugs can be lethal.

arthroscope projects images of the joint onto a screen and the surgeon can look for damage or make any repairs, such as removing damaged areas of cartilage or cartilage particles. Arthroscopy can help to alleviate the symptoms of osteoarthritis, but it cannot stop the progression of the disease.

There are other types of surgery performed for a variety of reasons, which may include:

- Preventing the joint from becoming deformed.

- Correcting an existing deformity.

- Removing part of the bone around the joint to allow for movement: This is called an osteotomy (which means cutting of a bone), and it is performed mostly on younger people, usually in a hip or knee. There are three types of osteotomy procedures: block osteotomy, in which a section of bone is removed; cuneiform osteotomy to remove a wedge of bone; and displacement osteotomy, when a bone is rebuilt to change the bone alignment on the areas that carry most of the body's weight. This may postpone joint replacement surgery for younger patients.

- Replacing a damaged joint with an artificial one. Artificial joint replacement is most commonly done on hips and knees, but can be done on wrists, ankles, and finger joints, as well. Artificial joint replacement is a very successful surgical procedure (see Chapter 10 for more information on artificial joint replacement).

- Immobilizing a joint, also called arthrodesis, or ankylosis. This is sometimes used to correct severe joint problems. The surgeon will make the joint permanently immobile through the use of metal or plastic screws or a special plaster. The AMA states that arthrodesis is used only when the pain from osteoarthritis is so severe that immobilizing the joint is an improvement. The procedure is usually performed on smaller joints, such as fingers or toes.

Looking down the road

There are new pain relief medications and treatments for osteoarthritis surfacing regularly. Nevertheless, it can take 20 years for research to prove that a new medication or treatment works. Scientists are currently working on:

- **Protease inhibitors:** Proteases are enzymes that break down cartilage. As the disease progresses, protease enzymes break down more and more cartilage. Scientists are working on developing a new class of drugs, called protease inhibitors, which will help to slow the action of these enzymes.

- **Regenerating cartilage:** It may sound like a scene out of *The X Files,* but scientists are experimenting with ways of regenerating our own cartilage in test tubes and transplanting the healthy cartilage back into our bodies. Chondrocytes are the cells that make cartilage, and the idea is to transplant them to a location where they can actually remanufacture the cartilage that was damaged, and then to transplant the new material into the affected area. Although this new treatment is progressing, it is not in general use yet.

- **Joint polymer:** A joint polymer, or polyurethane formulation, is implanted into a joint using minimally invasive techniques. According to studies, it can provide a smooth surface to restore joints in which the cartilage is degraded.

It's applied to the joint surface using arthro-scopy. The patient is reported to regain activity within 24 hours, but studies are still being conducted.

Living with osteoarthritis

How you must cope with osteoarthritis depends on the severity of the condition. If you are experiencing it in only one knee, you may have to make only min-imal adjustments to your lifestyle in order to cope with the pain. However, if your symptoms are severe, it is important to learn how to manage your pain and handle the interruptions of your flare-ups. Here are some tips (check Chapter 14 for more):

- Consider occupational therapy. An occupa-tional therapist is a trained and licensed health-care professional who can show you how your arthritis is affecting your lifestyle and suggest changes to help you cope. To find an occupa-tional therapist, ask your physician or a local hospital for recommendations. Your therapist will ask questions about hygiene, eating, clean-ing, cooking, driving, etc. The therapist also conducts a physical examination to check your range of motion, and may suggest splints or assistive devices, such as canes and walkers.

- Handy arthritis aids. There are bathtub grab bars, elevated toilet seats, knob turners, and extenders to help you reach out-of-the-way items. Assistive devices can help you with the tasks and challenges of living at home, or work-ing at your job.

- Eliminate your stress. Stress can cause a host of physical problems, including chronic fatigue, back pain, and headaches. Stress causes spasmodic pains in the neck and shoulders, musculoskeletal aches and lower back pain. Eliminating the stressors in your life may help reduce your joint pain.

■ Learn to say no. Know your limits. Doing too much for too many without taking time out for your own needs can only make your symptoms worse. Know when to say no and take a break. It's for your own good health.

Just the facts

■ Osteoarthritis is a fact of life for everyone eventually, but you can take steps to reduce your risk factors.

■ There are many treatments to reduce the pain of osteoarthritis, but lifestyle changes help too.

■ Over-the-counter medications like aspirin and acetaminophen can reduce pain temporarily.

■ Artificial joint replacement surgery is the most successful medical advancement in this century for arthritis.

Make sure you are not using the affected areas unnecessarily. For example, when I am tense I often clench my fists or hold myself in a stiff, unnatural position. It causes needless pain.
—Janet, 54

GET THE SCOOP ON...
What you may be feeling ▪ If you have the
'factor'? ▪ Updates on latest treatments ▪
Treating flare-ups

Rheumatoid Arthritis

Just looking at the gnarled, twisted, knobby fingers and swollen, misshapen joints of a person suffering from an advanced case of rheumatoid arthritis can be painful. Living with rheumatoid arthritis, however, can be debilitating. Rheumatoid arthritis is a disease that turns everyday tasks that are usually taken for granted—such as writing a letter, opening a door, dressing, and walking up the stairs—into barriers to independent living.

When your body rebels against itself

Rheumatoid arthritis is a disease marked by a failure of the body's autoimmune system—the system that, when it functions properly, is supposed to protect us from viruses and diseases. In rheumatoid arthritis, the immune system, in effect, turns on itself and attacks healthy joint tissue. This assault on the immune system causes inflammation of the synovium, a membrane that lines the joints. The affected cells respond to this inflammation by releasing an enzyme that can destroy the surrounding

65

Unofficially...
French impressionist painter Pierre Auguste Renoir, who lived from 1841 to 1919, suffered from severe rheumatoid arthritis for the last 25 years of his life. According to his grandson, painting was psychologically therapeutic for him. When he could no longer hold the brushes, he had others place them between his arthritic joints.

bone and cartilage. If the condition is left untreated, the affected joint can eventually lose its shape, resulting in pain, loss of movement, and possibly destruction of the joint.

If you suffer from rheumatoid arthritis, this battle is being waged inside your own body. Your symptoms—fatigue, soreness, stiffness, and aching—may creep up on you slowly, perhaps one joint at a time, and intensify.

Rheumatoid arthritis is a systemic disease, which means it slowly attacks all of your joints, but it doesn't stop there. The attack can charge on to your eyes, lungs, and heart. In some patients, rheumatoid arthritis can involve internal organs and cause serious damage, including inflammation of the blood vessels, called vasculitis. Vasculitis is a rare, serious complication that can stop the blood supply to tissues and cause tissue death.

Fortunately, over the past few decades, there have been many advances in the diagnosis and treatment of rheumatoid arthritis. One important advance is the discovery of the "rheumatoid factor" or the genetic factor that may cause rheumatoid arthritis. Scientists have also developed many effective medications that treat the symptoms of rheumatoid arthritis, and there are still many more to come.

It is never a good time to be diagnosed with a chronic illness, but if you're living with rheumatoid arthritis today, you have extensive options in medication and treatment available to you that were nonexistent just a few years ago. In this chapter, we will examine those treatments, the symptoms of rheumatoid arthritis, its possible causes, the most recent debate on using antibiotics to treat the condition, and how to reduce the pain and inflammation.

The risk factors of rheumatoid arthritis

Rheumatoid arthritis is not the most common form of arthritis, but when it strikes, it does not discriminate. Although it strikes most commonly in middle age, age really does not matter. There are more than 285,000 children and adolescents who suffer from a juvenile form of rheumatoid arthritis. Rheumatoid arthritis attacks both men and women, but women are affected two to three times more often, though researchers are not sure why. There are other risk factors for developing rheumatoid arthritis, including:

Genetic predisposition

Researchers believe that a virus may trigger rheumatoid arthritis in people who have the "rheumatoid factor,"—which is known in the scientific literature as RA factor HLA-DR4. This appears to be a genetic marker on the surface of the cells. If you are tested and found to have the rheumatoid factor, it means you may have an inherited tendency toward developing rheumatoid arthritis. The RF factor is an abnormal substance that occurs in the blood of about 80 percent of adults with rheumatoid arthritis.

If you are tested and found to have this genetic marker, it does not necessarily mean that you are going to develop the disease. Even if you have been diagnosed as having rheumatoid arthritis, it may help you to know that many patients experience periods of remission and might even feel as if they have been cured, at least for a short period of time. Although such periods of respite from the disease may be short lived, those with rheumatoid arthritis do their best to enjoy this time, using it to accomplish goals, such as exercising more or playing with

Unofficially...
Patients with rheumatoid arthritis make 7.8 physician visits annually—more than twice the national average for all individuals.

their children, activities that are more difficult during a flare-up.

Only about five percent of patients with diagnosed rheumatoid arthritis will progress to the advanced, most severe stages of the disease. If you are one of the unfortunate ones who have been dealt the more severe version of rheumatoid arthritis, you can at least be heartened by the knowledge that there are more options available to treat the flare-ups today than there were just a decade ago. An aggressive combination treatment plan consisting of medication, physical therapy, exercise, nutrition, and rest can force many painful flare-ups into remission.

Gender

According to the Arthritis Foundation, 1.5 million women have rheumatoid arthritis, compared with 600,000 men. Researchers are looking for answers as to why so many more women than men develop rheumatoid arthritis. In hopes of finding clues, they are studying the female and male hormones, particularly the female hormone estrogen. Interestingly, researchers have found that the symptoms of rheumatoid arthritis often improve or stop during pregnancy. Again, they are uncertain as to why, but results of one study suggests it may be related to differences in certain proteins between a mother and her unborn child. These proteins may help the immune system distinguish between the body's own cells and foreign cells. Such differences, the scientists speculate, may change the activity of the mother's immune system during pregnancy. Unfortunately, this nine-month breather is not permanent. Symptoms of rheumatoid arthritis usually return within a few months after the baby is born.

Minimizing the risks

You cannot totally eliminate the risks of developing rheumatoid arthritis. After all, you cannot change the fact that you are a woman or the fact that you have a genetic predisposition to rheumatoid arthritis. However, it is believed that you can lower your risk of developing the disease and help your body to reduce the severity of your symptoms.

Eat right

Good nutrition is one of the staples of good health, but preliminary research indicates a possible connection between foods rich in beta-carotene and a reduced risk of rheumatoid arthritis. A study from Johns Hopkins University suggests that a low level of beta-carotene in the blood may actually increase your risk of getting rheumatoid arthritis in the first place. Until further research has been completed, experts agree that eating right can make a difference, particularly if you eat foods high in beta-carotene such as:

- Sweet potatoes
- Pumpkin
- Carrots
- Cantaloupe

Nutritionists also suggest washing the fruit and vegetables down with water, another vital component of good health that washes away the toxins from your food.

The fish factor

You may want to add some fish to that healthy diet. Studies have shown that omega-3 fatty acids, polyunsaturated fat found in fish, may have an anti-inflammatory effect on the body. Omega-3 fatty

66

I was 30 when I was diagnosed with rheumatoid arthritis. My grandma had severe rheumatoid arthritis, and I didn't call my mom crying that I had it. Instead, I called her crying and said "I am going to have grandma's feet!" She had the ugliest twisted toes and feet, which were deformed from RA. I had nightmares about those feet when I was kid.
—Tina, 33

acids have already been touted as a way to decrease the risk of coronary heart disease. Now researchers believe that omega-3s also decrease the production of the tumor necrosis factor (TNF), a protein produced in high levels in rheumatoid arthritis patients. (More on tumor necrosis factor under "What are the causes of rheumatoid arthritis.")

Omega-3 fatty acid can be found in seafood, especially higher-fat fish, such as albacore tuna, mackerel, and salmon, or it can be taken as a dietary supplement. Some studies have shown that RA patients taking omega-3 supplements experienced significant reduction in pain, swelling, and an improvement in morning stiffness and fatigue. Research is still being conducted to see if omega-3 fatty acids can be used as an alternative to NSAIDs. The American Dietetic Association, however, states that fish oil supplements that contain omega-3 fatty acids are not recommended as a substitute for fish, or as a dietary supplement. The side effects of omega-3 fatty acids are minimal, consisting largely of nausea, flatulence, and diarrhea.

Exercise

Trying to exercise when you are suffering from the pain and inflammation of arthritis might seem impossible, but it just might be what you need to help combat the symptoms. Exercise creates strong bones, muscles, and joints and has been shown to decrease the symptoms of arthritis. Even exercising in small amounts has its benefits. Until recently, aerobic exercise was the only training routine recommended for optimal health benefits. Today, strength training, also known as resistance training, is recognized as an integral part of overall fitness.

In 1996, a Tufts University study found that even people with severe rheumatoid arthritis could safely increase their strength by roughly 60 percent in 12 weeks through a modest weight training program—or by performing resistance exercises. They were careful not to exercise during flare-ups and to rest whenever they felt joint pain, returning to strength training once a flare-up had receded.

What are the causes of rheumatoid arthritis?

The exact causes of rheumatoid arthritis are unknown, but many potential triggers have been tested, even mercury amalgam dental fillings, silicone breast implants, and root canals, although none have been proven to cause rheumatoid arthritis. More recently, the vaccination for hepatitis B and rubella (German measles) have come under scrutiny. Although some cases have been linked to both vaccinations, there has not been a clear determination if either one causes rheumatoid arthritis, or any other autoimmune disease.

What *has* been proven is that rheumatoid arthritis is a multifactorial disease, which means that there is more than one possible cause. Some of the causes that have already been proven include:

■ **Rheumatoid factor:** As we mentioned earlier, the rheumatoid factor is an abnormal substance that occurs in the blood of about 80 percent of adults with rheumatoid arthritis. This factor is a potential cause of rheumatoid arthritis and can be triggered by physical or environmental causes. Researchers are still looking into RF.

■ **Viruses:** Some researchers believe that a viral infection triggers the rheumatoid arthritis in people who already possess the genetic marker for the disease. Since rheumatoid arthritis is an autoimmune disease, it is believed that a virus can trigger the body's autoimmune response to fight the viral infection. However, when the infection is over, the autoimmune system does not stop its attack, but continues on to destroy the healthy cells.

■ **Tumor Necrosis Factor (TNF):** Recently, another cause of rheumatoid arthritis has been uncovered. TNF is a protein and chemical messenger, and it is an important part of the body's normal means to fight infections and injuries. During chronic illnesses, the body may overproduce TNF to harmful levels. In turn, these high levels can exacerbate the symptoms of a chronic illness, such as rheumatoid arthritis. Scientists are currently working on TNF blockers, or inhibitors, that can restrain the TNF before it causes any damage. Enbrel is the first such blocker approved by the FDA. Enbrel eliminates, or "soaks up" excess TNF before it can damage joints. Another potential TNF inhibitor, Remicade, is currently under FDA review. Enbrel is approved for use in combination with methotrexate (see "Treatment," below for more information).

The symptoms of rheumatoid arthritis

Like osteoarthritis, the symptoms of rheumatoid arthritis vary from person to person. You might experience mild pain that remains stable, while another person might have such a severe case that a joint or joints may be virtually destroyed, and only an artificial joint replacement can salvage any mobility. Fatigue; inflammation; and sore, stiff, aching joints are the most common symptoms of rheumatoid arthritis. Inflammation, which includes warmth, redness, and swelling of a joint, is a sign that the body is responding to an infection or trauma. Inflammation is a common symptom in rheumatoid arthritis, although not as common in osteoarthritis. To help diagnose rheumatoid arthritis, The American College of Rheumatology has established a list of symptoms that are found in rheumatoid arthritis patients:

- The presence of arthritis symptoms for longer than six weeks.

- The presence of nodules under the skin, called rheumatoid nodules, especially on the back of the elbows.

- Prolonged morning stiffness in the joints.

- Joint erosions apparent on an x-ray.

- Positive blood tests for the rheumatoid factor.

As mentioned before, the last item is not definitive: Twenty-five percent of people with rheumatoid factor never develop rheumatoid arthritis.

Treatment

Unfortunately, there is no cure for rheumatoid arthritis, but there are medications to help dull the pain, reduce the stiffness and inflammation, and help maintain normal joint function. Conventional therapy includes a combination of anti-inflammatory drugs and disease-modifying drugs that may slow the progression of the disease. How the body responds to treatment varies from person to person, so it may take time to find the right combination of treatments for you.

Watch Out!
Cigarette smoking significantly worsens the symptoms of rheumatoid arthritis and is considered to be a risk factor in triggering the disease. It is believed that smoking may cause abnormalities in the immune system of rheumatoid arthritis patients. Heavy smoking increases the white blood cell count and may increase the risk of infection.

Dulling the pain

Every year, new medications are introduced to reduce swelling and relieve pain and stiffness. It is important for you to know what is available to you and the side effects of using them. Later chapters will deal with these in greater detail, but here's a quick run down of what's out there.

- **Aspirin:** Aspirin reduces fever, relieves pain, and reduces swelling and inflammation. It is one of the more popular forms of treatment because it is cheap and effective, but it can also cause stomach and intestinal problems, such as ulcers and bleeding. Using large doses of aspirin over a long period of time can also cause blood clotting defects and liver and kidney damage. If you want to take aspirin, take a brand that has an enteric coating. This coating prevents the aspirin from releasing its contents until it reaches your intestines, thereby eliminating the stomach irritation. However, it may take longer for you to obtain pain relief. In some cases, aspirin may be prescribed at very high doses; if so, your doctor will monitor you closely for adverse side effects.

- **Acetaminophen:** If you cannot tolerate aspirin, the better choice for you may be acetaminophen, an aspirin-free pain reliever and fever reducer found in products such as Tylenol. Acetaminophen is safe when used as directed, but side effects can include severe anemia. Overdose can result in fatal liver failure. And combining acetaminophen with alcohol use can do the same thing.

- **Nonsteroidal anti-inflammatory drugs (NSAIDs):** The formal name for these medications is "nonsteroidal anti-inflammatory drugs, "commonly referred to as NSAIDs. Ibuprofen and naproxen are perhaps the best known of this class of medication. Over-the-counter versions of NSAIDs include Advil, Nuprin, Motrin, and Aleve.

These drugs are considered to be less toxic than aspirin, but can still cause gastrointestinal bleeding and kidney problems in some patients. NSAIDs slow the body's production of prostaglandins, substances that play a role in inflammation. They also carry some analgesic, or painkilling, properties. NSAIDs can be used if a patient does not respond to acetaminophen, but they must be carefully monitored for side effects, which include stomach trouble, gastric or duodenal ulceration, dizziness, skin rashes and ringing in the ears. To prevent some of the gastrointestinal irritation, it is recommended that NSAIDs should be taken with at least eight ounces of water. You are also advised not to lie down from 15 to 30 minutes after taking the drug.

▪ **Arthrotec:** If you are at high risk for gastrointestinal complications caused by NSAIDs and aspirin, there may still be relief in sight. Arthrotec, the brand name for diclofenac sodium, received U.S. marketing clearance from the FDA for osteoarthritis patients who are at a high risk for ulcers and other complications caused by NSAIDs. Arthrotec consists of an enteric-coated core that contains diclofenac sodium and misoprostol. There are side effects, including abdominal pain, diarrhea, and stomach upset, but it is believed that these side effects are not as great as those caused by NSAIDs. Women who are pregnant or plan to become pregnant should discuss the use of Arthrotec with their physicians, as this medication has been linked to birth defects.

- **Cox-2 Inhibitors:** Cox-2 inhibitors are another new class of painkillers that also promise to cause fewer gastrointestinal side effects than NSAIDs and aspirin. Cox-2 is an enzyme that has been found to cause the gastrointestinal distress associated with NSAIDs; a Cox-2 inhibitor stops this distress. Celebrex is the first Cox-2 inhibitor approved for sale by the FDA. Celebrex was compared to other NSAID products in several of these clinical trials by using endoscopes (a device to examine organs of the gastrointestinal tract) to determine the incidence of stomach and upper intestinal ulcerations following their use. These studies showed that patients taking Celebrex had a substantially lower risk of ulcers detected by endoscopy when compared to patients who took other NSAIDS.

The FDA is also currently reviewing Vioxx, another Cox-2 inhibitor. The makers of Vioxx are also touting the fact that Vioxx has fewer gastrointestinal side effects than NSAIDs. Additional information on Vioxx should be available some time this year.

Disease-modifying anti-rheumatic drugs (DMARDs)

Disease-modifying anti-rheumatic drugs work to slow or stop the basic progress of the disease. You may have to take them for several weeks or months before you notice any signs of improvement. The side effects can be substantial, so these medications are reserved for severe and progressive diseases. Some of the DMARDs include hydroxychloroquine, azulfidine, cyclosporine, sulfasalazine, azathioprine, and d-pencillamine. Here are a few more substances that may help slow the progression of the disease:

▪ **Gold salts:** It might sound like a folk remedy from the Old West, but gold treatments are DMARDs that have been used for years in the treatment of arthritis. The treatment consists of injections that contain real gold (in the form of a dissolved salt), but may have to be used for an extended period of time to gain the maximum benefit. There are minor side effects, including skin rashes and mouth ulcers.

You might also gain similar benefit by wearing gold rings. Studies have reported that gold rings may actually delay the progression of rheumatoid arthritis in the fingers on which they are worn.

▪ **Methotrexate:** Previously used as an anti-cancer medicine, this drug is now a commonly used DMARD for rheumatoid arthritis. It is used, with supervision, in low doses to suppress the system enough to reduce swelling and slow the damage and the progression of the disease. Methotrexate, prescribed by rheumatologists for decades, reduces the risk of death from rheumatoid arthritis complications by up to 50 percent, according to the American College of Rheumatology.

Methotrexate does have many side effects, including low white blood cell counts, gastrointestinal problems, sore throat, fever, nausea and vomiting. There are also many precautions and potential problems with the interaction of methotrexate and other medications.

▪ **Leflunomide:** Its brand name is Arava, and it is the first DMARD approved especially for rheumatoid arthritis treatment in more than 10 years. Leflunomide blocks the overproduction of immune cells that are responsible for most of the inflammation. Leflunomide has been shown to have positive results on early and advanced rheumatoid arthritis. Premenopausal women and pregnant women are advised not to take Arava, as it may cause birth defects.

▪ **Corticosteroids:** Corticosteroids are synthetic versions of the hormone cortisone and include prednisone and dexamethasone. Corticosteroids are generally prescribed for short-term relief for an intense flare-up to immediately reduce pain and inflammation and can be prescribed when patients do not find relief with other treatments. Unfortunately, while the relief is quick and dramatic, there can be serious side effects, including weight gain and thinning bones and skin. The shots are therefore reserved for just a few times per year.

Antibiotics and rheumatoid arthritis

The medical community is still undecided on whether rheumatoid arthritis is triggered by an infection and, therefore, would benefit from antibiotics. One side of the debate insists that if an infection were present, the bacteria would have presented itself and been removed during treatment with antibiotics; but rheumatoid arthritis is not curable. The other side believes that since research has shown that antibiotics have some effect in treating rheumatic diseases, it is enough to prove that an infection may be present and antibiotics may help.

In the meantime, the most talked about antibiotic treatment today is minocycline, a medication from the tetracycline family that was originally used to treat acne. The medication is believed to block metalloproteinases, enzymes that destroy cartilage inside joints. Minocycline also has anti-inflammatory properties and may suppress certain components of the immune system, the primary culprit in rheumatoid attacks. Rheumatologists are uncertain as to how the antibiotic works, but it appears to reduce the joint swelling and tenderness in some patients.

However, minocycline has not yet been approved by the FDA, and further research is needed to determine how the minocycline interacts with other drugs.

The final decision about antibiotic therapy for you should be made by your physician. It will not work for everyone and treatment must be individualized. Once the medication is stopped, the benefits stop too. Minocycline is a gentle medication that has only a few side effects, including splotches of dark patches on the skin, and dizziness.

If you are considering taking antibiotics for your arthritis, follow these precautions:

- Ask whether or not the medication should be taken with food or on an empty stomach.
- Know that antibiotics may cause yeast infections. Talk to your doctor.
- Avoid direct sunlight.
- Be aware that you may experience diarrhea.

Watch Out!
Do not continue taking anti-rheumatic drugs if you are pregnant or intend to become pregnant. These drugs can cross the placenta and affect the normal development of the fetus. As a result, they may cause birth defects. Also, if you are pregnant, notify your doctor before any x-rays are done or you take any medications.

Surgery

Like osteoarthritis, surgery is also a viable option for the damaged joints from rheumatoid arthritis, but your physician will first exhaust every other treatment possibility. Medications, physical therapy, exercise, and rest are commonly prescribed. Your doctor will work with different combinations to find the right one for your symptoms. However, your physician may consider you a candidate for surgery if your pain is at a severe, unacceptable level, if you have tried all other options of relieving your pain, or if your joint has been destroyed. Surgical options for arthritis pain include:

- **Osteotomy:** The surgeon may suggest repositioning the joint, called an osteotomy. This surgical procedure consists of removing damaged bone and tissue and restoring the joint to its proper position. Recovery time from an osteotomy can be lengthy, perhaps from 6 to 12 months, and it does not guarantee that the function of your joint will improve. Additional treatment may be necessary. Whether or not you need another procedure, and when that procedure will take place, will depend on the condition of the joint before the procedure.

- **Synovectomy:** Synovectomy is a type of surgery in which the synovium, the membrane lining the inside of a joint, is removed because it is inflamed and damaged by arthritis. The procedure was first introduced in 1923 as a hope of limiting further disease activity. Synovectomy is still performed, more commonly on finger and knee joints.

- **Arthroplasty:** Also called artificial joint replacement surgery, arthroplasty is a procedure that removes the diseased parts of the hip joint or knee and replaces them with new, artificial parts made of metal and plastic. Although knees and hips are common joint replacements, there are over 2,000 wrist implants and 7,000 hand and finger implants inserted each year, according to the *Journal of the American Medical Association*. There are also artificial joints for shoulders, fingers, ankles, and wrists.

A patient with a joint replacement should expect the joint to last for at least 10 to 20 years. You can maximize the odds for a successful replacement by staying at an ideal weight, exercising, protecting against infection, and avoiding impact sports.

There are risks to every operation, and joint replacement surgery comes with its own set, including dislocation, inflammation, phlebitis (blood clots of a vein), blood vessel and nerve damage, and possible revision surgery. If you are considering surgery, discuss all the options with your doctor and the risks involved.

> **66**
> Compensate by using your strongest joint and muscle to avoid joint stress.
> —The Arthritis Foundation
> **99**

Potential complications

Rheumatoid arthritis is a complicated disease. It can occur as an independent condition, or it can be associated with other diseases, such as:

- **Raynaud's phenomenon:** Patients with Raynaud's phenomenon have changes in the small blood vessels of the hands or feet when they get cold. Common symptoms include fingers that tingle, turn blue, and become stiff in response to the drop in temperature. The hands and feet do recover, but they are usually red and painful for several minutes afterward. There are medications that can help alleviate the symptoms, such as calcium channel blockers, but other side effects may limit what is prescribed. Instead, patients are advised to make adaptations to their lifestyle. For example, wear mittens or gloves and limit the exposure to the cold.

- **Sjogren's syndrome:** This is a chronic inflammatory disorder that includes dry mouth, eyes, and other mucous membranes. It is often associated with autoimmune disorders, such as scleroderma, rheumatoid arthritis, and lupus, but why it occurs is unknown.

Looking down the road

The medical community is always researching new methods of treatment, and hopefully a cure, for this debilitating condition that affects millions of Americans. Some of the recent research on rheumatoid arthritis includes:

- **Blood filtering:** A blood filtering machine has been invented that removes offending antibodies from the blood. It is currently awaiting final approval from the FDA. The machine, the Prosorbar Column, may be helpful with the most severe cases of rheumatoid arthritis.

- **Pain medications:** Remicade, from Centocor, could be approved for treating rheumatoid arthritis by this summer. Remicade was recently approved to treat Crohn's disease (an inflammatory bowel disease that has no, as yet, known cause).

Living with rheumatoid arthritis

There are ways to measure how much money is spent on rheumatoid arthritis research, and what monetary effect the disease has had on the economy. There are also ways to measure how many people are afflicted with this debilitating condition. But there is no possible means of measuring how this condition affects the individual lives of the people who suffer from it.

Rheumatoid arthritis takes a physical and emotional toll on its victims. First, it may be difficult to diagnose. You can be suffering from the early symptoms of the disease, but blood tests and x-rays may be frustratingly normal. Those suffering from rheumatoid arthritis may also have to combat various other emotional hardships, including:

- **Impacted personal life:** Coping with the stress of the burdens that your condition has put on the family. For example, perhaps you are no longer able to work and bring in a paycheck, or you must now depend on family members to help you dress, cook dinner, drive a car, or walk up the stairs. You may try to attempt to do these things yourself or avoid asking for help because you may feel that it is an imposition on another person. Even marriages suffer when a spouse has a chronic illness; the rate of divorce among these couples is much higher than couples without chronic illness.

- **Increased financial burdens:** As with any chronic illness, you'll be facing bills for doctor visits, medications, and assisted-living devices, such as walkers and canes. These bills can add up after time, but you may not be financially able to handle them. Approximately 50 percent of all rheumatoid arthritis patients must stop working within 10 years. Studies show that RA patients are more likely to have lost their jobs, retired early, or reduced their work hours due

Unofficially...
Comedienne Lucille Ball wasn't laughing when, as a teen, she suffered from rheumatoid arthritis. In her book, *Love, Lucy*, she describes the pain in her legs "as if they were on fire." Before the onset of this pain, she had incidents of pneumonia and fever, but no link to her arthritis was ever found. She tried horse serum and massage as miracle "cures."

to their illness. In severe cases, you may also be forced to leave your job and request disability payments.

- **Lowered self-esteem:** Rheumatoid arthritis is a cyclical condition, so you will probably face ups and downs. According to mental health experts, rheumatoid arthritis can destroy self-esteem as you lose the ability to be independent and self-sufficient. If the disease takes its long-term toll on the joints, you may even become repelled by your own changing physical appearance—at, for example, the misshapen joints that have replaced long, beautifully slender fingers. You are not alone with the way you feel. According to the Arthritis Foundation study of 500 rheumatoid arthritis patients, 81 percent were frustrated by the feeling of no longer being in control, and 32 percent could not get dressed when their rheumatoid arthritis was at its worst.

So how do you cope? There are many avenues of support and many ways to cope when you experience flare-ups in your condition. Here are just some tips. Check out Chapter 14, "Living Well with Arthritis," for more tips and suggestions. For now, here are a few that work:

- **Rest:** It is recommended that people with rheumatoid arthritis take a rest in the middle of the day. If your schedule permits it, find a quiet place where you can put your feet up, lay back, and take a short nap. Rest is vital to reduce swelling and joint stress and should be a planned part of your day, just as you would plan a business meeting or lunch with a friend.

When you are involved in an activity or project, you might not realize how much time has passed until you try to move. Stiffness and pain can take over your body, so make sure you change positions frequently, moving around a bit at least every two hours to prevent stiffness. If you sit too much, get out and take a walk. If you stand for prolonged periods of time, enjoy a few moments off your feet. Taking breaks and changing positions is also very important for people who keep their hands in one position for a long period of time, such as typists or craftspersons. Set an alarm clock if you must to remind yourself to take breaks.

- **Combat your depression:** Studies have shown that rheumatoid arthritis patients who have had even a single past episode of depression are at a greater risk for reporting pain, fatigue, and feeling disabled by their disease at a later date. Chronic pain and fatigue can lead to depression. Watch for these warning signs:

Bright Idea
Invest in a daily planner to help schedule all of your activities each day, and be sure to schedule in rest periods. This planner can also help you to spot what might have triggered a recent flare-up. For example, too much walking while window shopping at holiday time may have triggered a recent episode. Keeping organized will also eliminate stress and fatigue from overload.

  Excessive use of drugs or alcohol

  Personality changes; withdrawal from social activities

  Ongoing feeling of sadness

  Physical or verbal abuse

  Thoughts of suicide

Contact a doctor, hospital, psychologist, social worker or mental health center immediately if you feel you may harm yourself or others. And consider finding a support group or a therapist with whom you can open up about your feelings. Make sure your family members know how you feel, and talk to them about their feelings, too. After all, they are also feeling the effects of your condition.

■ **Eliminate stress:** Researchers have studied the link between stress and rheumatoid arthritis and determined that when you are stressed out, your arthritis flares up. When the subjects of these studies experienced stress, they were monitored to see if their stress increased their disease activity. In one-third of the patients, it did. Make sure you find out what is stressing you and make lifestyle changes to eliminate or reduce the stress factors in your life. Even small changes can make a big difference.

Acceptance is key

Okay, this isn't always an easy one, but promise yourself you are going to work on it. By accepting the fact that you are going to have bad days, it is emotionally easier to cope with them when they arrive. Here are some words of wisdom from one rheumatoid arthritis sufferer:

> Rheumatoid arthritis is a hideous beast that takes you down roads luckier people never have to travel. I spent eight days in the hospital—including Christmas Eve and Christmas Day. It would be rather easy to wallow in self-pity and bemoan my lot in life right now, but it is quite clear to me there is an abundance of things to be thankful for that drown out any depression I may feel. Rheumatoid arthritis is a never-ending battle and the patient must never lose his will to fight it. Self-pity and depression are intruders on the battlefield. Rid yourself of them as quickly as they appear.
>
> —Carol, 43

Just the facts

- Rheumatoid arthritis is a chronic disease, with periods of flare-ups and remissions.

- The chronic inflammation of rheumatoid arthritis can cause permanent joint destruction.

- The "rheumatoid factor" is a genetic marker that can be found in 80 percent of patients with rheumatoid arthritis, but this does not mean you will develop the condition.

- Treatment for rheumatoid arthritis is individual, but includes a combination of education, rest and exercise, joint protection, medications, and possible surgery.

GET THE SCOOP ON...
The mysterious illness ▪ Risk factors ▪
18 points of pain ▪ The sleep connection ▪
Pain reduction

Fibromyalgia

Fibromyalgia is a syndrome that affects your bones and joints; it is as frustrating as it is debilitating. You often wake up from another restless night's sleep with stiffness in your muscles, and widespread pain in your body that lasts hours past your morning cup of java. Your muscles are aching, throbbing, and burning, and you are convinced that arthritis is taking over your bones. You are so exhausted that just taking care of your basic daily responsibilities takes every ounce of energy that is left in your weary body, and you have no strength left for anything else. Even if you try to take a nap, or two, or three, it fails to energize or refresh you.

The frustrating mystery of fibromyalgia

You are getting frustrated as friends, family members, and co-workers find it difficult to believe that you are sick when, from the outside, you appear normal and healthy. Your symptoms may wax and wane for months and can include recurring headaches, dizziness, and diarrhea. Your social life is strained

89

and your job is on the line because you just cannot keep up. You have also used up all of your sick days for your many doctor appointments and tests.

Cynics insinuate that you are just suffering from stress; that you just need more sleep, more exercise, a change in your diet, or a simple daily vitamin. No one understands how, despairingly, you have dragged yourself from doctor to doctor and been subjected to test after test and, even years later, you still do not have a name for your malady.

After some time, you might even start to believe your critics. Maybe this is all in your head and maybe you are a hypochondriac. Does this sound familiar? If so, rest assured that you are not a hypochondriac and your symptoms are most definitely not just in your head. Your symptoms are real and your condition does have a name: fibromyalgia syndrome, or FMS.

This chapter may finally help guide you to the right diagnosis. If you have already been diagnosed with fibromyalgia, it may be comforting to you to know that millions of Americans have fibromyalgia and that there are methods of coping with the pain and techniques that you can use in your everyday life to help handle flare-ups.

Solving the mysterious illness

According to the American College of Rheumatology, between three and six million Americans, mostly women, suffer from fibromyalgia, but this disabling condition was only identified less than two decades ago.

Over the years, many theories have circulated about what is now known as fibromyalgia. Some of these speculations included:

- The belief that it was a connective tissue disease, like scleroderma. As a result, fibromyalgia was once named fibrositis, which means inflammation of the fibrous tissues. It was later discovered, however, that there was no inflammation involved in fibromyalgia.

- The belief that it was associated with rheumatoid arthritis and Lyme disease. The symptoms of fibromyalgia mimic the symptoms of many autoimmune diseases, including rheumatoid arthritis and Lyme disease, so it was believed to be linked to these conditions. Fibromyalgia has also been called rheumatism, myalgia, and pressure-point syndrome, and has been linked to other conditions such as hypothyroidism and lupus, but researchers have proven that fibromyalgia is not arthritis, although the symptoms are closely related.

- The belief that it was a psychological disorder. Rheumatoid arthritis and osteoarthritis can be diagnosed through blood tests and x-rays, but there are no diagnostic tests that can detect fibromyalgia. As a result, physicians once thought it was a condition of the mind, not the body.

Although research has shown that patients who suffer from fibromyalgia do suffer from psychological traits such as depression, there are physical findings of tender points in the body, as well as pain and stiffness. Depression and other psychological disorders are now considered to be a response to having fibromyalgia, not a cause of it.

Thanks to this research, in 1987 the American Medical Association finally recognized fibromyalgia

Unofficially...
Fibromyalgia was first described by William Balfour, a surgeon at the University of Edinburgh in 1816, but it was never given an official medical name until the late 1980s. Since Balfour's description, the medical community had struggled to properly name this puzzling illness that plagues millions, but leaves physicians confounded when the afflicted patients fail to show any abnormalities on x-rays or in laboratory tests.

"
Listen to your
body. If it tells
you to stop and
lie down, do so.
This took me a
long time to
learn. Like other
FMS patients who
are very active, I
didn't want to
accept this dis-
order. Learn to
pace yourself
and not overdo
things, even if
you are feeling
good that day.
Once a flare-up
starts, no one
can predict how
long it will last.
—Betty, 65
"

as a true physical illness and a major cause of dis-ability among Americans. Unfortunately, however, in many cases it has not changed the lengthy amount of time between the initial onset of symp-toms and the final diagnosis. Physicians will still attempt to exhaust all other possibilities before ren-dering a diagnosis of fibromyalgia. This lengthy process may be annoying and frustrating to some patients, but unless tests are being performed repeatedly or unnecessarily, a complete physical can help to rule out other potential illnesses.

What is fibromyalgia?

Now that you know what fibromyalgia isn't, the med-ical community is still unsure exactly what it is and what causes it. What is known so far is that fibromyal-gia is a painful musculoskeletal condition that originates in the muscles and soft tissues that sur-round the joints, but not directly in the joints.

Fibromyalgia is a very individualized syndrome. Not everyone will experience all of the symptoms. Some patients undergo a constant battle with many symptoms, while others have some symptoms that fluctuate from day to day. Some patients suffer from mild pain, tenderness, and fatigue, while others can suffer from severe pain and disabling fatigue. The most commonly reported symptoms of fibromyalgia include:

- Widespread aches and pains, which usually occurs on both sides of the body and must be present for at least three months to be classified as FMS.

- Stiffness that occurs mostly in the morning, and is located around the areas of the neck, shoul-ders, back, and hip areas. Stiffness can also be triggered when a person has been idle in one position, perhaps sitting at a computer, for too long

- Headaches.
- Dry mouth.
- Cold hands and feet.
- Facial pain.
- Irritable bowel syndrome, which includes abdominal pain, bloating, constipation or diarrhea.
- Swelling in soft tissue, not the joints.
- Costochondraglia, or muscular chest pain where the ribs meet the chest bone.
- Muscle spasms.
- Psychological symptoms, such as depression, anxiety and mood swings.
- Memory and occasional speech difficulties.
- Tender points throughout the body.

In 1990, the American College of Rheumatology developed 18 painful and tender points in the body that are usually present in a patient with fibromyalgia. You must have pain in at least 11 of the 18 criteria points in order to be diagnosed as fibromyalgic. These tender points include:

- The base of the skull.
- Midway between the neck and shoulder.
- The muscle over the inside shoulder blade.
- 2 cm below the elbow joint.
- Upper outer buttock.
- Hip bone.
- Above knee on inside.

- Lower neck front.
- Edge of upper breastbone.

Diagnosing fibromyalgia

X-rays, blood tests and other diagnostic tools that doctors regularly use to diagnose arthritis are not effective in diagnosing fibromyalgia. However, physicians rely on these tests to help them rule out other possible illnesses or conditions. Once other conditions have been eliminated, doctors rely on the results of a physical examination, and the 18 tender point test for confirmation of fibromyalgia.

What causes fibromyalgia?

The exact cause of fibromyalgia is not yet known, although researchers have gotten closer in finding certain triggers for the condition. They include:

- **Genetics:** Genes are pockets of information that determine your characteristics from height and eye color to what disease predispositions you may have inherited. Studies have shown that fibromyalgia occurs within several members of one family, which may indicate a genetic link. Studies have also shown a link between fibromyalgia and patients who have a family history of alcohol or depression.

- **Injury or trauma:** It is believed that an injury or trauma to the body may affect the central nervous system and the level or intensity of pain.

- **Muscle metabolism:** Lack of blood flow to the muscles may cause muscular fatigue and decreased muscular strength. Again, this may trigger additional FMS symptoms.

- **Substance P:** Researchers have found that patients with fibromyalgia have twice as much

Timesaver
You may visit many doctors before an accurate fibromyalgia diagnosis is made. To save time, maintain a journal that includes your symptoms, the name and phone number of each doctor you have seen, the dates, the tests that were run, and the results. This will also save you money on repetitive testing. The doctor will also have a paper trail of your history.

Substance P, a chemical substance which helps nerve cells communicate with one another. This extra Substance P may produce increased levels of pain sensitivity. Researchers are studying the brains of fibromyalgia patients, searching for answers as to why they experience severe pain. They have begun focussing on this Substance P. They believe that patients with fibromyalgia have a decreased blood flow to the areas of the brain that deal with pain, which prevents oxygen from circulating properly and leads to fatigue. This fatigue may trigger FMS symptoms. In addition, reduced blood flow means less Substance P circulates in the brain, possibly stimulating it's overproduction, and thus a hypersensitivity to pain.

■ **Somatomedin C:** Somatomedin C is a substance that is needed by the body to produce human growth hormone (HGH). The release of HGH is controlled mainly by the central nervous system and occurs in bursts. More than half the total daily amount is released during deep sleep. Since patients with fibromyalgia do not sleep well, it is believed that there is not enough somatomedin C released during this time. As a result, a lack of somatomedin C causes a lack of HGH production and a subsequent lack of proper muscle tissue repair. Again, this leads to fatigue, which can trigger the FMS symptoms.

■ **Psychological disorders:** Although research has ruled out stress and other psychological disorders as causes of fibromyalgia, scientists still believe that the psychological symptoms such as trauma and stress can cause flare-ups of the condition.

- **Serotonin:** Serotonin is a natural body chemical that plays a role in constricting blood vessels, stimulating smooth muscles, and transmitting impulses between nerve cells. When the level of this chemical is low, it is believed that this triggers widespread aches, pain, and fatigue.

- **Fatigue factor:** Researchers are looking at chemicals that may be produced in the body that cause severe fatigue and "brain fog."

- **Sleep disturbances:** Researchers are studying the impact which poor sleep has on your body and its connection to fibromyalgia. For example, imagine how you feel having one bad night's sleep. The next day, you are usually tired and cranky because you did not sleep well. Now imagine experiencing that feeling night after night for months on end. Researchers believe that this poor sleep can trigger FMS symptoms.

Researchers are also studying stage four, or the deep period, of sleep. It has been shown that patients with fibromyalgia have abnormal brain waves during deep sleep and it is believed that these abnormal brain waves may trigger symptoms. Insomnia and sleep apnea—when a person stops breathing during sleep for short periods of time—are also thought to be triggers for fibromyalgia, although these theories have not yet been proven.

Who gets it?

Fibromyalgia primarily occurs in women of childbearing age, but children, the elderly, and men can also be affected. The American College of Rheumatology states that fibromyalgia is a very common syndrome that afflicts up to five percent of the American population. They also believe that this percentage would be much higher if the patients who were misdiagnosed or undiagnosed were correctly categorized.

Fibromyalgia can strike anyone at any age, but it most frequently affects women between the ages of 20 and 40, although the reasons are not currently known.

Treatments

There are no known cures for fibromyalgia. Instead, patients are encouraged to treat their muscular and joint pain and make lifestyle changes to reduce the risk of flare-ups.

Establish a regular sleep routine

We just discussed the link of poor sleep to fibromyalgia. Although it has not been medically proven, physicians still recommend that patients establish a regular sleep routine to reduce the risks of flare-ups. For example, you try to go to sleep at 10 p.m., but one night you stay up late watching a movie, another night you are having trouble falling asleep, and on a third night you are up late talking with a friend. As a result, your normal sleep pattern is erratic and you are overtired by the end of the week. Then you try to play "catch up" by sleeping late on the weekend.

Wishful thinking, but this does not work. Your body cannot store extra sleep to be used at a later time when you need it. Also, even though you may feel refreshed after sleeping late on a Saturday, your body cannot catch up on sleep you have already lost. In addition, this erratic and disturbed sleep pattern can cause a flare-up in your symptoms. Since research has already made a connection between deep sleep and FMS, the established sleep pattern is important to help control your symptoms. Make sure you plan a regular sleep schedule and stick to it.

Tricyclic antidepressants: a medication that can help

To help improve your sleep, especially the deep sleep phase, physicians will prescribe tricyclic antidepressants. Tricyclic antidepressants are also called CNS depressants, which means that they slow down the central nervous system and may possibly cause drowsiness. Antidepressants are more commonly used as a treatment for depression, but tricyclic antidepressants can boost serotonin levels. Higher serotonin levels can relieve muscle pain and spasms and help relieve some of your symptoms. Commonly prescribed antidepressants include:

- **Amitriptyline:** This drug is more commonly known by its brand name Elavil or Endep. Amitriptyline improves the quality and the depth of sleep, rather than the mood. Amitriptyline is usually taken before bedtime and should be taken with food.

- **Fluoxetine:** You may know this by its brand name, Prozac. In the last 10 years, Prozac has been touted as the cure-all for depression. In one drug trial, a low dose of Prozac in the morning with a low dose of Elavil at night has been shown to effectively reduce symptoms of fibromyalgia in some patients. Prozac works by affecting the chemical messengers within the brain called neurotransmitters. It is possible that an imbalance in these neurotransmitters is the cause of depression. Some FMS patients may not be able to tolerate Prozac; ask your doctor about alternatives.

Watch Out!
Know one knows just why, but pregnancy seems to relieve symptoms of fibromyalgia. It is believed that the hormonal changes of pregnancy act to suppress these symptoms. However, if you are thinking of becoming pregnant or think you may already be pregnant, contact your doctor immediately. Not all medications for fibromyalgia are safe for an unborn child.

Watch out for side effects

All medications can cause some side effects, but how you react to a particular drug is highly individual. It cannot be stressed enough that you should inform your physician and pharmacist about all of the medications you are currently taking so they can check for potentially fatal interactions when medications are combined. If you experience any side effects from any medication, contact your physician immediately. Some side effects can be a simple nuisance, such as dry mouth, and may require an adjustment of the dosage. Other side effects may be fatal. Some minor side effects of the tricyclic antidepressants when taken by themselves include:

- Blurred vision.
- Drowsiness.
- Dizziness.
- Weight gain.
- Dry mouth.
- Fuzzy headedness.

Do not stop taking these medications suddenly unless instructed by a physician. Some antidepressants, such as Prozac, need to be slowly weaned from your body.

Dulling the pain

Every year, new medications are introduced to relieve muscular and joint pain. It is important for you to know what is available to you and the side effects of using them. Over-the-counter medications are available to help relieve the symptoms of fibromyalgia including:

- **Aspirin.** Aspirin reduces fever and relieves pain and is one of the more popular forms of treatment, because it is inexpensive and

> 66
> At first I felt a little sad but I thought of how much worse it could be and accepted it. I know that it is not a debilitating disease and it is not going to get worse so whatever discomfort I have I can deal with it.
> —Patricia, 63
> 99

effective. However, it can also cause stomach and intestinal problems, such as ulcers and bleeding. Using large doses of aspirin over a long period of time can also cause blood clotting defects and liver and kidney damage. If you want to take aspirin, take aspirin that has an enteric coating. An enteric coating means that the aspirin will not release its contents until it reaches your intestines, thereby eliminating the stomach irritation. However, it may take longer for you to obtain pain relief. In some cases, aspirin may be prescribed at very high doses; if so, you must be closely monitored for side effects.

■ **Nonsteroidal anti-inflammatory drugs.** Nonsteroidal anti-inflammatory drugs, commonly referred to as NSAIDs, are commonly prescribed to decrease inflammation and relieve the pain of arthritis. NSAIDs include ibuprofen and naproxen with over-the-counter versions such as Advil, Nuprin, Motrin, and Aleve. However, while these medications may be helpful in treating arthritis, they should be used sparingly when treating fibromyalgia symptoms. NSAIDs can help to alleviate the muscular and joint pain of fibromyalgia, but inflammation is not a symptom of fibromyalgia. These drugs may also cause gastrointestinal bleeding and kidney problems in some patients.

■ **Acetaminophen.** If you cannot tolerate aspirin, the better choice for you may be acetaminophen. Acetaminophen is an aspirin-free pain reliever and fever reducer, such as Tylenol. Acetaminophen is safe when used as directed, but side effects can include severe anemia. Overdose can result in fatal liver failure.

- **Cyclobenzaprine.** Otherwise known by its brand name Flexeril, this is a muscle relaxant that relieves pain, muscle spasms, stiffness, and discomfort, but does not affect muscle function. This medication is prescribed for short-term use, approximately 2 to 3 weeks.

- **Corticosteroids.** Corticosteroids are synthetic versions of the hormone cortisone and include prednisone and dexamethasone. Corticosteroids, such as Lidocaine, are generally prescribed for short-term relief for an intense flare-up to immediately reduce pain and inflammation. Corticosteroids are normally recommended when patients do not find relief with other treatments. Unfortunately, while the relief is quick and dramatic, there can be serious side effects, including weight gain, and thinning bones and skin. These injections are reserved for just a few times per year.

The exercise option

How can you think of exercising when you hurt so badly? It is not easy, but even if you can find the energy to walk or add some exercise to your day, it may help to relieve some of your symptoms. Exercise reduces joint pain and stiffness and increases flexibility, muscle strength, and endurance. Do not rush into an exercise program or expect quick results. You might do more damage to your joints than good. Take your time and be patient and you will eventually see results. Start with exercises that you can do in a sitting position and slowly work up to a full, more intense routine.

If you exercise regularly and correctly, you should be able to increase your program without becoming totally fatigued just from the exercise.

Watch Out!
Fibromyalgia patients should avoid prescription tranquilizers and sleeping medications from the benzodiazepine group. According to research, these medications suppress deep sleep and can intensity your FMS symptoms the next day. Alcohol and narcotics may also have the same affect and combining them can be deadly.

Bright Idea
Pace yourself
when you
exercise—
overdoing it is a
bad idea. Too
much exercise in
a short period of
time can cause
injury and strain,
increasing your
pain. Ease into
your exercise
routine, and
although you
may experience
mild soreness at
first, it will stop
once you've
established a
regular routine.

There are three types of exercises that you should be doing to help your body stay healthy and strong and help to reduce the severity of your symptoms. They include:

- **Range-of-motion exercises:** These stretching exercises help to maintain normal joint movement, and maintain or increase flexibility. These are gentle stretching exercises, done daily, that keep joints mobile and prevent stiffness.

- **Aerobic or cardiovascular exercises:** Aerobic exercise improves cardiovascular fitness and helps to burn calories and control weight. Weight control is important because excess weight puts pressure on your joints. Aerobic exercise also helps the blood to circulate properly throughout the body. This is important to get oxygen and nutrients to all the organs, tissues, and muscles, especially the heart. Aerobic exercise also strengthens blood vessels, increases blood supply and decreases the risk of cardiovascular disease, which can narrow and weaken blood vessels. When muscles do not get an adequate supply of blood, they can cramp. Good blood circulation is also needed to help tissues heal after injuries. Examples of aerobic exercise include:

    Walking

    Running

    Cycling

    Rowing

    Stair climbing

- **Strength training:** The more strength muscles have, the more they can lift. This does not mean that you need large muscles to be strong. While some muscles or groups of muscles may be stronger than others, overall strength is important. It enhances the ability to perform activities, such as carrying baskets of laundry, and taking care of the lawn and garden. Strength training, also known as resistance training, is recognized as an integral part of overall fitness. Examples of strength training exercises include free weights and machines, isometrics, elastic bands, step straps, and using your own or a partner's weight against your own body weight.

Avoiding stress

Stress itself does not damage joints or tissues, but when you are stressed out, your muscles tighten up, especially your neck, shoulders, and back, and can contribute to your pain and trigger flare-ups of fibromyalgia. There are many ways that you can control your stress, but in the long run you need to experiment and find something that works for you. Some ideas include:

- Listen to your body. Hungry? Overtired? If you need a healthy snack or a nap—do it.

- Relax! Take at least 15 minutes a day to watch TV, read a magazine, or participate in a favorite hobby.

- Avoid alcohol and drugs. These crutches will only create problems and increase anxiety.

- Get organized. Buy an appointment book and write yourself little "remember" notes to alleviate the distress of being unprepared and the brain fog of FMS.

Moneysaver
Exercise gyms can be expensive; instead, ask for a free visitor's pass. Try the equipment and visit at different times to see how busy the club is. Do not fall for slick salespeople offering you discounts and incentives during your visit. Instead, make an educated consumer decision. Walking can also get your heart pumping and tone your muscles—and it's free.

- Recognize any source of stress besides FMS: job, family, or schedule. Eliminate unnecessary burdens and learn how to say no.

- Find a support group. Talking with people who also have fibromyalgia and understand your pain can reduce irritation.

- Laugh! Watch a funny video, crack up with pals. What better way to enjoy life and eliminate aggravation?

- Have a massage. Scientific evidence supports the theory that touch promotes healing and relaxation, but the best part of a massage is how good it feels.

A wide variety of techniques are available to you, including the most common Swedish massage and Japanese "finger pressure" Shiatsu. Massage not only alleviates physical and mental irritations but also improves circulation and skin elasticity, and decreases the recovery time from fatigue and muscle soreness.

Eat better to feel better

Good nutrition cannot cure the symptoms of fibromyalgia, but sensible eating provides your body with the proper nourishment to be strong and healthy. Quick sugar fixes, such as a candy bar, or your morning and afternoon cups of coffee only give you short bursts of artificial energy. When the burst is over, these stimulants actually leave you feeling more sluggish than before. Then you need another short burst and this continues the cycle of poor eating and a poorly nourished body. Healthy eating should provide enough of the right nutrients for strong muscles and bones. Talk with your physician before taking vitamin supplements.

Moneysaver
Many fibromyalgia syndrome sufferers use massage as treatment to help with the pain, discomfort, and stress. Massage therapists who are affiliated with a doctor's office may be covered by your medical insurance or only cost a minimal copay. Ask your physician and health insurance provider to see if you are eligible.

Learning to cope with fibromyalgia

The proper diagnosis of FMS can take years. In the meantime, it may be difficult, whether or not you are an otherwise active person, to accept the fact you now have physical limitations. Even after the diagnosis is in, you may still feel frustrated when you are told that there is no cure, pharmaceutical treatment is minimal and that you are an integral part of the pain management process.

People who suffer from fibromyalgia are eager, if not desperate, to find something to help them ease the pain. As a result, they may try anything that claims to reduce the pain they are feeling. Some items, such as hot and cold packs, acupuncture, meditation, and tai chi are relatively safe. Other products, however, can be dangerous to your health. If someone is touting a product that you have not heard about before as a cure for FMS, think twice before trying it. Ask your physician for more information about the product and whether or not it may help your symptoms. In the meantime, to help you cope with your symptoms:

- Find a support group. Others with FMS can relate to how you feel. If you need help finding a support group, or want to start one in your area, check with your local hospitals. (See Chapter 15 for additional information on support groups.)

- Find a support network. This does not have to be a formal support group, but a small circle of friends or family members who understand and believe what you are feeling.

- Accept help. Handling a debilitating condition by yourself is not always easy. When someone wants to help, learn how to say yes.

Moneysaver
Many doctors are still not familiar with fibromyalgia. Question your physician about any tests that are being performed more than once and thoroughly explain your symptoms. If your physician does not seem very sympathetic about your symptoms or is performing unnecessary testing, consider changing doctors.

■ Just try to cuddle. Fibromyalgia in itself doesn't affect the sex drive, but medications may impair it, leaving couples frustrated. In addition to medications, patients with fibromyalgia are usually so fatigued, depressed, and in pain that the idea of being touched and exerting energy is not appealing. Cuddling or just spending time together in different ways can help during flare-ups.

Looking down the road

Research is still needed to better understand what causes fibromyalgia. Studies on these possible causes and diagnostic methods are currently underway:

■ **Cortisol:** Researchers think low levels of this hormone may trigger FMS symptoms.

■ **Adrenal gland:** Researchers are studying the regulation of the adrenal gland, which manufactures cortisol and regulates metabolism.

■ **Magnetic resonance imaging:** Researchers are studying this tool as a means of diagnosing fibromyalgia.

■ **Sex hormones:** It is thought that since fibromyalgia affects more women than men, it may be related to a woman's level of estrogen. Researchers are also studying levels of testosterone, the male sex hormone, which is also responsible for muscle strength.

Just the facts

■ Fibromyalgia is a real condition that affects the musculoskeletal system.

■ It may take quite some time to diagnose your fibromyalgia. In the meantime, try coping techniques.

66

When my fibromyalgia flares up, I just slow down and get through the day the best I can. It is typical for doctors to tell a woman it is stress, but I read an article about this lady who had a disease that mimics arthritis, but it could have described me. Then I knew it wasn't in my head.
—Joan, 48

99

- Change your lifestyle to minimize your risks of flare-ups.
- There are currently no cures for fibromyalgia, but there are medications to help decrease your pain and discomfort.

GET THE SCOOP ON...
The "other arthritises" ▪ Whether you are at
risk ▪ Minimizing your odds ▪ How to lessen
the hurt

Related Disorders

Chapter 6

As you learned back in Chapter One, arthritis is not the name of a single disease, but rather a general term used to describe more than 100 different rheumatic diseases that affect the joints, muscles, and connective tissues of the body. We have already discussed two of the most commonly occurring and generally recognized types of arthritis: rheumatoid arthritis (discussed in Chapter Four) and osteoarthritis (detailed in Chapter Three). In Chapter Five you learned about one syndrome that is often misunderstood and diagnosed as possible arthritis: fibromyalgia. It is impossible to discuss all of the 100 different types of arthritis in one book and provide you with a thorough explanation of each. This chapter, however, will tackle some of the more common arthritis-related disorders.

The dangers of self diagnosis

If you are tempted to use this chapter to help you diagnose your symptoms, don't. It is impossible to diagnose your symptoms simply by reading a book because there are many different causes for the many different types of arthritis. For example, the chronic arthritis associated with Lyme disease is a bacterial infection that is acquired through the bite of an infected tick. Transient arthritis, on the other hand, is a form of arthritis that is caused by a viral infection such as the mumps, German measles, hepatitis B, or parvovirus infection. And reactive arthritis can start in the aftermath of another infection, such as a sexually transmitted disease.

This is just a small portion of the types of arthritis that you may have. While this chapter can educate you and help to *direct* you to the right diagnosis, it is up to you to make an appointment with your physician and have a thorough physical. Your physician is the only person who can accurately diagnose your symptoms and recommend appropriate treatment. Your symptoms are unique and only he can help determine what you may have. This is important because some symptoms may be shared by more than one type of arthritis. By attempting to diagnose yourself, you could be missing a vital piece of information that may cost you valuable time once you attempt to obtain the right medical treatment for your specific condition.

Because the symptomology of many forms of arthritis can be confusing, trying to diagnose your symptoms may require that you make several visits to specialists, including:

- Endocrinologists—physicians who specialize in hormonal and metabolic disorders.

- Rheumatologists—physicians who specialize in joint and muscle disorders.

- Otolaryngologists—also known as ENTs, these physicians specialize in ear, nose, and throat disorders.

■ Neurologists—physicians that specialize in nervous system disorders.

Finding the appropriate specialist (or specialists) is an important part of diagnosing your symptoms. It may take time to rule out the many other disorders that mimic your particular "flavor" of arthritis before your physician can determine exactly what you may be suffering from. This chapter will help you to become familiar with some of the more common related disorders to arthritis and learn how you may be at risk for them—as well as how you can try to minimize your likelihood of developing the conditions, if you *are* at risk. If you do not find mention here of the specific disorder that concerns you, turn to Appendix B, "Resources," for a list of the many organizations dedicated to dealing with arthritis and arthritis-related disorders. There you will quite likely to find a group or society that can directly address your specific concerns.

Connective tissue diseases

As mentioned earlier, the word "arthritis" simply means an inflammation of the joint—a condition that gives rise to symptoms such as swelling, stiffness, tenderness, redness, and warmth. Remember that inflammation is a sign that your body is fighting an injury or infection. Your body responds to this infection or injury (also called a trigger) by sending tissue-building cells to the affected area. Chemical messengers called cytokines and prostaglandins are also sent to the site. These substances take control of the healing process and enhance the cell growth.

Once the healing has taken place, the inflammation should subside. But this is not always the case. The antibodies that were sent to fight the virus or bacteria can suddenly turn against their host and

Bright Idea
If you need to see several doctors in pursuit of a diagnosis, keep a log of the physician's name, the date of your exam, tests performed, and their results. Include phone numbers and addresses so that you can retrieve copies of test results, if necessary. This eliminates unnecessary testing and creates a paper trail that will help your doctor diagnose your condition.

begin to destroy the healthy cells in the area. This is called an autoimmune disorder—a disorder in which the body engages in battle with its own healthy tissues. An autoimmune disorder can cause joint pain, rashes, and, if severe enough, internal organ damage as well. Rheumatoid arthritis is one well-known example of a connective tissue disease that also involves an autoimmune disorder. Others include myositis, Raynaud's phenomenon, scleroderma, Ehlers-Danlos syndrome, Sjogren's syndrome, lupus erythematosus, and vasculitis.

Raynaud's phenomenon

Raynaud's phenomenon occurs when the blood vessels of the hands, feet, ears, and nose constrict in response to exposure to the cold. This is not to be confused with the normal feeling of being cold that you might experience, for example, when you have forgotten to wear gloves on a winter day. Raynaud's phenomenon is much more severe, causing the hands or feet to first turn white, then blue, and finally a painful red. There are two kinds of Raynaud's phenomena: primary and secondary. Primary Raynaud's phenomenon occurs by itself, with no underlying diseases or medical problems. Most patients with primary Raynaud's are between 15 and 40 years old and 75 percent them are women. Secondary Raynaud's syndrome is more rare, but the patient will also have an underlying disease or condition that causes this phenomenon, such as scleroderma.

There is no known cause of Raynaud's phenomenon, but it is believed to be triggered by exposure to cold or emotional stress. The attacks are also linked to other types of arthritis, such as rheumatoid arthritis and scleroderma.

Treatment for Raynaud's phenomenon will depend on whether or not the disorder is an underlying condition of another disease (such as rheumatoid arthritis or scleroderma) or a disease on its own (in which case it would be called primary Raynaud's). Nonmedical treatments may include protecting the body from exposure to cold temperatures, controlling stress, and exercising. Medications can also be used to help minimize the discomfort of an attack and to try to prevent further attacks, but this is not always successful. These medications may include:

- Calcium-channel blockers that dilate the small blood vessels and relax the muscles.

- Alpha blockers that prevent the constriction of blood vessels.

Scleroderma

Scleroderma is an autoimmune disease of the connective tissue that affects 150,000 people in the United States alone, according to the Scleroderma Foundation in Danvers, Massachusetts. The name "scleroderma" comes from two Greek words and means "hard skin"— thickening of the skin is one of its most common symptoms. There are two types of scleroderma: localized, which is manifested by a few affected spots on the skin; and systemic, which can damage the internal organs such as the lungs, heart, and kidneys. In severe cases, scleroderma can be fatal, but the American College of Rheumatology reports a 60 to 70 percent five-year survival rate. Other symptoms of scleroderma include:

- Raynaud's phenomenon.

- Swelling of the hands and feet.

Unofficially...
Here is another reason to quit smoking. Smoking has been shown to cause the skin temperature to drop, which may lead to an attack of Raynaud's phenomenon and can aggravate breathing difficulties in ankylosing spondylitis. If you have a problem quitting, consult your physician for a medically approved method. It's for your own good health.

- Pain and stiffness of the joints.

- Joint contractures: an abnormal condition wherein a joint is bent and will not move. The contracture is caused by shortening and wasting away of muscle fibers. A person suffering from scleroderma may trigger a contracture by keeping the affected joint in one position in an effort to minimize the pain of inflammation.

- Calcinosis, or small calcium deposits around the elbows, knees, or fingers.

- Difficulty swallowing.

- Sjogren's syndrome, characterized by dry mucous membranes.

- Weakness, weight loss, and muscle aches.

Tests to diagnose scleroderma include:

- Erythrocyte sedimentation rate (ESR).

- Rheumatoid factor tests.

- Anti-nuclear antibodies tests.

There is no known treatment that will reverse or stop scleroderma. However, there are topical creams and moisturizers that can be used to help soften the skin. Medications, including DMARDs and NSAIDs, are available to help minimize the pain and discomfort of scleroderma. Another promising treatment is minocycline, an antibiotic that has been used to treat cancer and has now been shown in studies to stop the progression of scleroderma. More research is needed, however, and minocycline has not yet received FDA approval for this use.

Ehlers-Danlos syndrome

Ehlers-Danlos syndrome could be described as the opposite of scleroderma. Ehlers-Danlos syndrome is a genetically inherited connective tissue disorder that leads to stretchy, fragile skin. Joints become loose and unstable and can easily be dislocated or are easily extendible. It is believed to be caused by a defect in the connective tissue and by faulty collagen. Ehlers-Danlos syndrome can trigger early onset of osteoarthritis.

Sjogren's syndrome

Sjogren's syndrome is an incurable autoimmune disorder that affects between 2 million and 4 million Americans; nine out of ten of whom are women. In this autoimmune battle, the moisture-producing glands (tear ducts and salivary glands, for example) are attacked by the body's own immune system and destroyed. The syndrome can continue to damage vital organs, or it can go into remission. Symptoms include blurred vision, recurrent mouth infections, swollen salivary glands, hoarseness, difficulty swallowing, and eating. Skin, nose, and vaginal dryness are also possible symptoms. There are two types of Sjogren's syndrome:

- Primary, which affects the eyes and salivary glands without the presence of another connective tissue disease.

- Secondary, which accompanies a disease that affects the connective tissue. Fifty percent of those with Sjogren's syndrome have this type.

Treatment for Sjogren's includes moisture replacement therapy, NSAIDs, corticosteroids, and DMARDs to slow the progression of the disease.

Lupus

Lupus is another autoimmune disease that causes inflammation of the skin, joints, blood, and kidneys. Between 1.4 million and 2 million Americans have lupus; 90 percent of them are women. Some forms

Unofficially...
Charles Kuralt, the legendary CBS-TV newsman, was diagnosed with lupus shortly before his death. His obituary states that he died of complications from the disease. Mary McDonough, an actress best known for her role as Erin, one of the numerous children on *The Waltons*, has also made her battle with lupus public.

of lupus are mild, while others can be life threatening. The causes of lupus include:

- Defective genes.
- Overproduction of hormones.
- Faulty clearing of antibodies after an infection.

The symptoms of lupus include painful, swollen joints; muscle pain; fever over 100°F; extreme, prolonged fatigue; skin rashes; chest pain upon deep breathing; unusual hair loss; pale or purple fingers or toes in response to cold or stress; and sensitivity to sunlight.

There are three different types of lupus:

- Drug-induced lupus can be traced to the use of drugs such as hydralazine (a high-blood–pressure medication), procainamide (use to treat irregular heartbeats) and isoniazid (a tuberculosis drug). Symptoms usually fade when the medication is stopped.

- Discoid lupus is limited to only the skin. Symptoms include a rash on the face, neck, and scalp. This type of lupus does not affect internal organs.

- Systemic lupus erythematosus. Systemic means that it effects the entire body, not just one part. So systemic lupus erythematosus, or SLE, can affect almost any organ or system of the body. Ten percent of lupus patients have this type.

The first sign of SLE is often arthritis (in the most general sense of the term—joint inflammation). Some other early symptoms include a red rash over the nose and cheeks, weakness, fatigue, and weight loss. In addition, SLE sufferers develop an increased sensitivity to light, a fever, skin sores on the neck, and hair loss. SLE can also cause anemia and swelling of the blood vessels of the kidneys, the linings of the lungs, and of the abdomen. SLE can lead to kidney failure and severe nerve disorders.

Treatment includes topical steroid medication that can be applied to the rash, and NSAIDs to ease pain and swelling in the joints. Physicians generally recommend lifestyle changes as well, such as avoiding fatigue and stress, and protecting yourself when in direct sunlight.

More members of the arthritis family

Of course, we've only seen the tip of the arthritis iceberg so far. There are a great many other diseases and syndromes characterized by joint inflammation. Here are some more that fall into that broad basket of illnesses known as arthritis.

Gout

Years ago, gout was considered the disease of those who were rich enough to afford luxurious dining and drinking. Today, however, gout is recognized as a distinct medical condition caused by an excess of uric acid in the body. The association of gout with wealth, therefore, wasn't so far off the mark—only the wealthy could afford the rich sauces, fatty foods, and vast quantities of alcohol to wash them down (a prime recipe for the overproduction of uric acid if there ever was one). Fortunately, those who suffer from the wrath of gout attacks today have treatment options and medication that can help prevent future painful attacks.

Most gout attacks occur in the big toe, but gout can also attack the fingers, elbows, knees, and ankles. The attacks appear rapidly and are extremely painful. An episode may include swelling, discoloration, fever, and an acute tenderness to the

Unofficially...
Gout has the unique distinction of being one of the most frequently recorded medical illnesses throughout history.

affected area. The attack may last hours or days; it may be self-limited or need treatment.

The causes of gout include a genetic predisposition, obesity, weight gain, alcohol intake, high blood pressure, abnormal kidney function, and the use of certain drugs that increase the uric acid in the body.

The most reliable test for diagnosing gout is arthrocentesis, a joint-fluid test that detects the presence of uric acid crystals in the fluid. X-rays can be helpful and may show uric acid crystal deposits, as well as bone damage if you have suffered from repeated inflammations.

When treating gout, the most important goal is to prevent future attacks. You can do this by:

- Eliminating from your diet foods that trigger gout attacks, such as organ meats (liver, kidney, sweetbreads, and brains); meat gravies and extracts; sardines; anchovies; herring; mackerel; scallops; and most wild game. The following foods are only allowed once per day: meat, fish, poultry, dried beans and peas, asparagus, mushrooms, cauliflower, and spinach. See Chapters 12 and 13 for more details on how healthy eating and exercise can help minimize your risk of gout attacks.

- Eliminating alcohol.

- Decreasing uric acid levels in your system. Medications such as probenecid and sulfinpyrazone can effectively decrease uric acid blood levels by increasing its into the urine. Allopurinol (zyloprim) lowers the blood uric acid level by preventing uric acid production.

- Drinking plenty of water, up to two quarts per day, also helps to increase the excretion of uric acid.

Medications for gout include NSAIDs such as colchicine, probenecid, sulfinpyrazone and allopurinol. Allopurinol has the added benefit of helping to prevent kidney stones. Corticosteroids, such as prednisone, are powerful anti-inflammatory agents that are injected directly into the inflamed joint to reduce painful swelling.

Inflammatory bowel disease

Also known as ulcerative colitis, inflammatory bowel disease is a disorder that strikes the large intestine and rectum. Symptoms include watery diarrhea that contains blood, mucus, and pus, and severe intestinal pain, fever, chills, anemia, and weight loss. It is believed that chronic inflammation ultimately damages the bowel and then the infected bacteria travels through the bowel wall to the bloodstream, causing problems in other areas of the body. Inflammatory bowel disease can lead to joint and connective tissue disorders, including tendonitis, arthritis of the hip and of the outermost joint of the finger, and ankylosing spondylitis.

Treatment includes sulfasalazine, corticosteriods, immunosuppressives, and NSAIDs.

Lyme disease

Lyme disease was first identified in Lyme, Connecticut, in the early 1980s. It was, at the time, a mysterious condition that was ultimately traced to infection through the bite of deer ticks infected with the spirochete bacterium *Borrellia burgdorferi*. In 1982, the medical community began a serious effort of tracking incidents of Lyme disease, and in 1996 a total of 16,461 cases (from 45 states and the District of Columbia) were reported to the Centers for Disease Control and Prevention in Atlanta. This was a 41 percent increase from the 11,700 cases

It's hard to remember to take medication when I feel good, but it's a mistake not to. The pain can be so intense that it can make you cry. You can't walk, or put your shoes on. Pay attention to the doctor. Change your diet, stop drinking alcohol, or whatever is recommended. The pain isn't worth that beer or that piece of meat or shrimp.
—Chris, 35.

Watch Out!
The Lyme-bearing tick is very small, and it's easy to suffer a bite before you have a chance to spot the insect on your skin. Three shots of the new vaccine, LYMErix, are needed for the best protection against Lyme disease, but having at least two—the original and a booster—is advisable if you are planning a trip to a Lyme "hot zone."

reported in 1995 and a 32-fold increase in reported cases since tracking began in 1982.

Lyme disease includes flulike symptoms such as inflammation, swelling, chills, fever, headache, discomfort, Bell's palsy, and a ring-like rash at the point of initial infection.

One of the most significant advances this century has been the development of a vaccine to prevent Lyme disease. LYMErix is now available and considered very effective at preventing Lyme disease.

While treatment for Lyme is now readily available, it's only helpful in avoiding Lyme-related complications (like chronic arthritis) if you seek medical attention early. Unfortunately, many of the early symptoms of Lyme are easy to ignore or to confuse with something else, like a touch of the flu. If you are suffering the general symptoms listed above and you know you've been in a Lyme "hot zone" (much of New England or the Mid-Atlantic states), it's advisable to request a blood test that specifically looks for Lyme disease. This is one arthritis trigger that can actually be deactivated if you get treatment before the damage has been done.

Myositis

Myositis is a swelling of muscle tissue, usually of the involuntary muscles, such as the heart and lungs. Myositis can range from a skin lesion to a fatal disease. Causes of myositis include injury, infection, and invasion by parasites. Unfortunately, the same medications that are used to treat myositis can also cause the condition to become life threatening. This is because the medications act to reduce the effectiveness of the body's immune system, thereby making the patient more susceptible to infections.

There are different forms of myositis, including:

- Polymyositis, which affects the shoulders, upper arms, and thighs.

- Dermatomyositis, which affects the skin.

- Inclusion body myositis, which affects and the muscles of the hands and feet; it usually affects older individuals.

- Drug-induced myositis, which may develop after taking certain prescription medications. Symptoms generally disappear within weeks to months after the drug is discontinued.

- Occular myositis, which affects the eye muscles.

- Viral myositis, which is caused by a virus; symptoms usually disappear on their own.

Treatment includes NSAIDs and corticosteroids such as prednisone, prednisolone, medrol, deltasone, cortisone, and others.

Osteoporosis

Osteoporosis is a condition commonly associated with aging. Its prevalence alone is enough to justify that it be given separate treatment here. The word literally means "porous bones"—bones that deteriorate with age and become increasingly susceptible to the risk of fracture (commonly to the hips, spine, and wrists). As we mentioned in Chapter One, bones are not static materials, but living tissue that is constantly reformed in a process called remodeling. Every day, old bone is removed and replaced with new bone tissue. But with the age, this natural process slows, resulting in the common bone disease that we know as osteoporosis.

Bones continue to increase in density and calcium content until you reach your 30s, at which point you probably have attained your peak bone mass. Afterward you may either maintain this mass or begin to lose calcium yearly, but you rarely can increase bone density. For women, this loss of bone density is commonly accelerated during menopause, when their bodies cease to produce estrogen, a hormone required to improve bone strength.

Watch Out!
Forget the steroids. Men who use steroids are at a high risk for losing large amounts of bone within the first year of their use—as much as 10 to 20 percent. Men who use steroids also have a 50 percent chance of developing osteoporosis than men who don't.

When more bone is lost than is replaced (a process known as demineralization), your bones will begin to weaken and lose density. When the bone loses sufficient density, you face eminent danger of suffering a fracture. One out of two women over the age of 50 suffers an osteoporosis-related fracture during her lifetime. And, as you age, your risk for such fractures increases. In the U.S. alone, 10 million individuals, including men, already have the disease, and 18 million have low bone mass, placing them at risk for osteoporosis.

In extreme cases of osteoporosis, even everyday activities can assume danger: fractures can result from such low-stress activities as lifting a bag of groceries or taking a minor fall. Some women, fearful of fractures, eliminate many seemingly innocuous activities from their daily lives. Their fear is well-founded—complications from these fractures are a major killer of women. But such a fear-based response can lead to increasing isolation and a severely restricted lifestyle.

Prevention

The good news about osteoporosis is that research suggests it may be preventable and controllable. Regardless of age, you can lower your risk for the disease by eating right, consuming enough calcium, and performing weight-bearing exercises.

- Eating right. Eating a diet rich in the nutrients that help your bones stay strong—calcium, magnesium, vitamin D, phosphorus, soy-based foods, and fluoride—should be your first step toward stopping or slowing the process of osteoporosis.

■ Calcium. Increasing your calcium intake through dietary supplements is another very helpful and effective way to reduce your rate of bone loss.

■ Exercise. Lifting weights and performing other weight-bearing exercises are good ways to encourage your body to improve your bone density. And without regular strength training, muscles become weak. As you age, a total of 10 to 12 percent of your strength is lost, particularly between the ages of 30 and 65. This can result in a decreased activity level, increasing your risk of injury to muscles and bones, and presenting an increased risk of bone diseases such as osteoporosis and arthritis.

■ Reduce your caffeine and alcohol intake. According to the National Osteoporosis Foundation, caffeine may actually increase calcium loss. Alcohol and caffeinated products act as diuretics and alcohol may interfere with the body's absorption of calcium.

■ Quit smoking. Smoking causes a 5 to 10 percent loss of bone mass and has been shown to decrease estrogen levels, which can lead to bone loss.

Diagnosing osteoporosis

If you are at risk for developing osteoporosis, you should have a dual-energy x-ray absorptiometry test (DEXA or DXA). This is a type of bone-density test that measures bone loss in your spine and hips. It can detect even a one-percent bone loss. DEXA is a

Unofficially...
The Bone Mass
Standardization
Act was intro-
duced in
Congress to
ensure that the
cost of bone
mass measure-
ment is covered
under Medicare
and that stan-
dards for cover-
age are clear and
consistent for
anyone
with medical
insurance.

short, 10 to 15 minute procedure that consists of lying on a padded platform while a mechanical wand-like device scans your body. The amount of radiation from this procedure is only a fraction of what is used in a chest x-ray. (Not all insurance carriers cover DEXA tests, so check with your carrier before having the test done.)

You are at risk for osteoporosis if you:

- Have a family history of osteoporosis and related bone fractures.
- Had early or surgically induced menopause.
- Are a smoker and heavy drinker.
- Have an overactive thyroid gland.
- Are anorexic.
- Have scoliosis (abnormal curvature of the spine).
- Have a history of stress fractures.
- Are of Asian or Northern European descent.
- Have not had a child.
- Lead a sedentary lifestyle.

Treatment

The first goal of any osteoporosis treatment is to prevent bone breakdown. Medications that prevent bone breakdown are called bisphosphonates and include alendronate, (Fosomax), edidronate (Didronel), and calcitonin.

Fosamax is approved by the FDA for treating osteoporosis. It is well tolerated with few side effects. Didronel, an FDA-approved drug used for treating Paget's disease, has yet to receive approval for use in treating osteoporosis. It has been shown, however, to increase bone density in postmenopausal women. Calcitonin is a naturally occurring hormone secreted by the thyroid gland that also inhibits abnormal bone resorption. It has also been shown to prevent bone loss, but only of the spine.

Hormone replacement therapy (HRT) is another popular treatment for the prevention of bone loss. HRT supplies estrogen to women in menopause, but medical experts are still arguing over HRT's possible role in increasing the risk of breast cancer. Estrogen should not be taken by women at a higher risk for developing breast cancer, or by those who are already suffer from the disease.

A final roundup of arthritis family members

As you can see, the family of arthritis-related diseases is large and varied. Here are a few more of the better-known "family members." Keep in mind that, although we've covered a great many of arthritis's manifestations, there are still dozens more that we haven't the space here to discuss.

Paget's disease

Earlier in this chapter (and in Chapter One) we discussed the remodeling process of the bone. Paget's disease accelerates this process, causing bone pain, weakness, and soft, abnormal bones. Paget's disease usually affects middle-aged and older people, and may cause deformed skull bones, arthritis, fractures, bowing of the limbs, and possible hearing loss.

The cause of Paget's disease is unknown, but studies have shown that it may be caused by a virus that affects the bone; there is also a suspected genetic link.

Treatments for Paget's disease include:

- Bisphosphonates, drugs that inhibit abnormal bone resorption. Three bisphosphonates approved in the U.S. for treatment of Paget's

> **❝**
> I'm at risk for breast cancer—my mother had it—so I won't take estrogen. I'd rather do what I can without medications. My preference is to watch my diet and exercise as much as I can. That gives me my best chance to avoid osteoporosis.
> —Pat, 63
> **❞**

disease include alendronate sodium (Fosa-maxr), etidronate disodium (Didronelr), and pamidronate disodium (Arediar).

- Calcitonin, a hormone secreted by the thyroid gland that also inhibits abnormal bone resorption.

- Surgery may be necessary to repair any fractures. Total joint replacement of the hips and knees may be necessary, but is usually reserved for the severe cases, when other methods of treatment are no longer effective.

Polymyalgia rheumatica

According to the National Institute of Arthritis and Musculoskeletal and Skin Diseases, polymyalgia rheumatica is a rheumatic disorder that is associated with moderate to severe muscle pain and stiffness in the neck, shoulder, and hip area. The symptoms are most noticeable in the morning. The cause of polymyalgia rheumatica is still unknown, but immune system abnormalities and genetic factors are suspected. The NIAMSD states that since polymyalgia rheumatica is rare in people under the age of 50, it suggests it may be linked to the aging process. Treatment for polymyalgia rheumatica includes corticosteroids and NSAIDs.

Soft-tissue rheumatic syndromes

Soft-tissue rheumatic syndromes are manifested by a swelling of the connective tissues that surround a joint, but these syndromes are not actually classified as arthritis. They may be caused by injury, strain, or inflammation of tendons or ligaments. Soft-tissue rheumatic syndromes include:

- Plantar fasciitis: ligaments in the sole of the foot become inflamed, leading to pain on the bottom of the heel when you walk.

- Achilles' tendonitis: The Achilles' tendon is located at the back of the ankle and may become inflamed.

- Carpal tunnel syndrome: nerves pass through the carpal tunnel on the front of the wrist into the hand. Pressure on these nerves can lead to pain, numbness, and tingling.

Treatment for soft-tissue rheumatic syndromes include taking rest breaks from repetitive activities, wearing splints, applying heat or ice, NSAIDs, steroid injections, and sometimes surgery. For example, surgery for carpal tunnel syndrome divides the carpal ligament so that it no longer presses on the nerve.

Spondyloarthropathies

Spondyloarthropathies is generic term for conditions that cause chronic inflammation of the spine, including ankylosing spondylitis, Reiter's syndrome and arthritis associated with inflammatory bowel disease. These conditions also share one possible cause, the genetic factor HLA-B27.

Ankylosing spondylitis: This condition generally affects the bones of the spine, which may grow together and cause extreme back stiffness and inflexibility. Ankylosing spondylitis and juvenile ankylosing spondylitis can also affect the eyes, heart, lungs, and kidneys. Other symptoms include:

- Shortness of breath.

- Inflammation of the breast bone, or costochondritis.

- Tendonitis.

- Inflammation of the eye, or iritis.

- Kidney failure, in severe cases.

Even though the condition sounds debilitating and painful, almost all people who have ankylosing spondylitis can expect to lead normal and productive lives. This condition rarely causes full disability. Treatment includes exercise, NSAIDs, corticosteroids, and DMARDs.

Reiter's syndrome: Reiter's syndrome is thought to be caused by a viral or fungal infection that affects the ankles, feet, and lower back joints. It may begin with unexplained diarrhea and a mild fever. Other symptoms include sores and arthritis that often last after the original symptoms have been resolved. Antibiotics are used to treat the infection and NSAIDs are used to relieve the pain and swelling in the joint. The patient often recovers, but arthritic symptoms may continue off and on for many years.

Psoriatic arthritis: Psoriasis is a skin disorder that causes patches of red, thick, dry, silvery scales that are seen on the arms, scalp, ears, and pubic area. Psoriasis can lead to psoriatic arthritis, a chronic joint inflammation. Ten percent of patients who have psoriasis also develop inflammation of the joints. In some patients, the arthritis actually precedes the skin condition. Symptoms of psoriatic arthritis include "pitting" of the nails, wherein the nails look a bit like the surface of a thimble; joint stiffness; inflammation of the tendons (tendonitis); additionally, inflammation of the chest wall and of the cartilage around the breastbone which can cause chest pain, as seen in costochondritis. Treatment for psoriatic arthritis includes NSAIDs, corticosteroids, and DMARDs.

Reactive Arthritis: Reactive arthritis starts after an infection such as gastroenteritis or a sexually transmitted disease. It affects one or two of the larger joints such as the ankles or knees, and may also involve the lower back. It usually disappears after the infection has been treated.

Looking ahead

Scientists are still researching all members of the arthritis family. Recent studies include:

- New treatments for connective tissue diseases, including plasmapheresis, the removal of plasma from blood cells; photophoresis, the use of a drug activated by ultraviolet light; and penicillamine, a drug that interferes with collagen production.

- Fetal cells connection to scleroderma. Scientists have discovered that fetal cells may affect the development of scleroderma in women. Fetal cells that enter a woman's blood stream during pregnancy can still be detected up to 27 years later. These fetal cells may have the potential to form a wide variety of immune cells.

- Stem cell transplantation. Stem cell transplantation is currently being studied as a treatment for lupus. While this transplantation removes unhealthy cells, there is a 5 percent chance that the stem cell transplant may cause the patient to die. Because of this, the procedure is only performed on patients who have exhausted all other forms of treatment.

- Vitamin D and psoriatic arthritis. Recent studies suggest that a form of vitamin D may help psoriatic arthritis patients.

66
When flares take hold, I keep in contact with my doctor, ask friends to visit, and try to listen to my body when it says 'rest' I pray that my new medication will work soon. My children suffer too. A mom who can't drive has it tough in suburbia where there are no buses—especially when your children are 8, 10, and 12 years old.
—Michelle, 39
99

Just the facts

- There are too many types of arthritis to try to diagnose your own symptoms.
- If you have symptoms, contact your doctor immediately.
- Symptoms of different types of arthritis may overlap.
- Physicians may need to rule out some forms of arthritis to determine what type you may have.

GET THE SCOOP ON...
Risk factors ▪ Reducing risk ▪
Pain management ▪ The parent's role

Juvenile Arthritis

More than 40 million Americans, or one in six people, have been diagnosed with arthritis. Arthritis is a general term used to describe more than 100 different rheumatic diseases that affect the joints, muscles, and connective tissues of the body. One of the most common myths surrounding arthritis is that it is a disease associated only with aging. This is simply not true. Arthritis can strike anyone, even infants. Approximately 285,000 children in the United States have juvenile arthritis, and more than 70,000 of them have juvenile rheumatoid arthritis, the most common form.

This chapter will help you learn about juvenile rheumatoid arthritis. You will learn whether your child is at risk, how you can ease the pain, tips to help cope, and where to turn when you need support.

Arthritis and children, an overview

Children can develop many of the same disorders in the arthritis family that afflict adults, including systemic lupus erythematosus (SLE), juvenile

131

Unofficially...
Rest easy moms and dads. If your child has a knuckle-cracking habit, the most damage your child has done is to annoy you. Cracking knuckles will not lead to arthritis. The cracking sound is simply caused by a rapid release of the synovial fluid inside the joint, not by any real damage done directly to the joint.

dermatomyositis, ankylosing spondylitis, Reiter's disease, psoriatic arthritis, scleroderma, inflammatory bowel disease, and Lyme disease (see Chapter 6 for more detailed information on these conditions).

Most likely you are a parent or caregiver who is reading this chapter to learn more about your child's symptoms and illness, and to discover what you can do to help your child. If your child is exhibiting symptoms that fit into any one of the 100 types of arthritis, the most important part of your job is to obtain an accurate diagnosis and, of course, appropriate medical treatment. Depending on how old your child is, he or she may not be able to communicate well to you the symptoms that he or she is experiencing, so you must be observant—delaying proper medical care may prevent your child from receiving crucial treatment to stop the progression of the disease and reduce the accompanying pain.

Taking care of a child who is diagnosed with any illness or disease can be hard work. As a parent or caregiver, you may be responsible for administering medications, making doctor appointments, and supporting your child through painful flare-ups. Most likely, you are also trying to sort through your own emotions, especially when you see your child in pain. Juvenile arthritis does not just affect a child physically; it can have profound emotional effects as well. And living with a chronically ill child can have an impact on other members of the family who do not have arthritis. Educating yourself, your family, and especially your child as much as possible about arthritis is the first step in learning how to cope with the disease.

Juvenile rheumatoid arthritis (JRA)

In addition to the "adult" forms of arthritis that children can get, there's one form that they can call their very own. This is juvenile rheumatoid arthritis, a condition that affects about 70,000 children in the United States alone. Juvenile rheumatoid arthritis is very similar to adult rheumatoid arthritis. It is a disease marked by a failure of the body's autoimmune system—the system that, when it functions properly, is supposed to protect us from viruses and diseases.

As you'll recall from Chapter 4, in rheumatoid arthritis the immune system, in effect, turns on itself and attacks healthy joint tissue. This assault on the immune system causes inflammation of the synovium—the membrane that lines the joints. The affected cells respond to this inflammation by releasing an enzyme that can destroy the surrounding bone and cartilage. If the condition is left untreated, the affected joint can eventually lose its shape, resulting in pain, loss of movement, and possibly the destruction of the joint.

When children are affected with juvenile rheumatoid arthritis, they have not yet reached the age where they have achieved full bone development. Unfortunately, the chronic inflammation of the arthritis may have a damaging impact on the growth center of the bone. If the condition is left untreated long enough for the growth center of the bone to be damaged, the child may stop growing. If no damage has occurred, the child will continue to grow once the arthritis is under control. This means that early diagnosis and timely treatment are key.

Fortunately, children with juvenile rheumatoid arthritis may outgrow the illness, whereas adults with rheumatoid arthritis will usually have

Bright Idea
If your child is old enough to explain his or her symptoms to the doctor, rehearse the visit before you go. Make sure your child explains exactly where the pain is located and try to pinpoint exactly what kind of pain or other symptoms he or she is having.

symptoms for the rest of their lives. According to the National Institute of Arthritis and Musculoskeletal and Skin Diseases (NIAMSD), more than half of all children with rheumatoid arthritis will outgrow their symptoms.

But a simple diagnosis of juvenile rheumatoid arthritis is not enough. There are three distinct types of JRA, each of which carries its own constellation of symptoms. In the sections that follow you'll learn about each of these types of JRA in greater detail.

Polyarticular JRA

The term "polyarticular" refers to the fact that five or more joints are affected by arthritis (the prefix "poly" means "many"). Those who are diagnosed with polyarticular juvenile rheumatoid arthritis will usually test positive for the rheumatoid factor. Thirty percent of all children with juvenile rheumatoid arthritis have polyarticular disease; girls are more prone to this type than boys are, but it is not understood why. Some children with polyarticular disease have a special antibody in their blood, called IgM rheumatoid factor. This factor may lead to a more severe form of the disease, similar to adult rheumatoid arthritis.

Polyarticular juvenile rheumatoid arthritis affects the small joints of the fingers and hands. It may also affect the knees, hips, ankles, and feet, and it usually affects the same joint on both sides of the body. Other symptoms include:

- Low fever.
- Rheumatoid nodules: These are bumps under the skin, usually found on the back of the elbows.

- Long-term complications such as a slowed growth.

Pauciarticular JRA

Pauciarticular juvenile rheumatoid arthritis means that four or fewer of the joints are affected by arthritis (the prefix "pauci-" means "few"). This form of arthritis usually affects the large joints, and only one side of the body. Pauciarticular juvenile rheumatoid arthritis may also cause other disorders, such as iridocyclitis, which is an inflammation of the eye; iritis, which is an inflammation of the iris; and uveitis, which is an inflammation of the inner eye, or uvea. Children who develop iridocyclitis are also at risk for chronic eye inflammation. Treatment for iridocyclitis includes eye drops that will dilate the pupil and keep scars from forming, as well as decrease the inflammation in the eye tissues.

According to the NIAMSD, many children outgrow this type of arthritis by the time they are adults; but the eye problems associated with the disease can plague them for life, and joint symptoms may return.

Systemic JRA

As you learned in Chapter 6, a systemic disease is one that affects the entire body, not just one particular area. Systemic juvenile rheumatoid arthritis, also known as Still's disease, is a form of the disease that affects both the joints and the internal organs. It affects 20 percent of all children who have juvenile rheumatoid arthritis, and it affects boys and girls equally. Symptoms of systemic juvenile rheumatoid arthritis include:

Timesaver
Maintain a journal to document your child's symptoms and take it to appointments. It will help the doctor recognize patterns or underlying symptoms that may contribute to your child's condition. Include when and where your child complained of symptoms or when you noticed any physical changes in your child. List any allergies, current medications, and a family health history.

- High fevers that usually start in the late afternoon or evening. These fevers can reach 103° or higher, but may drop to normal within just a few hours.

- Chills and shaking.

- A light pink rash.

- Anemia, or a low red blood cell count. This may lead to fatigue, dizziness, headache, insomnia, and pale skin.

- High level of white blood cells.

- Enlarged lymph nodes.

- Long-term complications may include slowed growth.

Less commonly seen symptoms may include:

- Inflammation of the outer lining of the heart, also called pericarditis.

- Inflammation of the heart.

- Inflammation of the lungs, also called pleuritis.

Sometimes the symptoms of juvenile rheumatoid arthritis may subside for a time. This phenomenon is known as a remission, and it can last for months or years. All three types of juvenile rheumatoid arthritis may also share additional symptoms, including:

- Joint damage.

- Joint stiffness.

- Muscle and other soft tissue weakness.

- Joint erosion—In severe juvenile rheumatoid arthritis, the long-lasting inflammation may damage the surfaces of the joint. This may cause pain and limit the range of motion of the affected joint.

- Joint contracture—When a child holds a painful joint in the same position for a long period of time, the muscles can stiffen up and become weak. The tendons may also tighten up and shorten, causing what is called a joint contracture. The joint will not move. This may have to be treated with surgery.

Diagnosing JRA

A pediatrician is the medical specialist who normally takes care of a child, but when a child has arthritis, your pediatrician may call in the assistance of a pediatric rheumatologist, an ophthalmologist (eye doctor), an orthopedic surgeon, and/or a physiatrist—a physician who specializes in physical medicine—as well as an occupational therapist.

Diagnosing arthritis in children is not always easy. Children can frequently compensate well for loss of function and may not complain of pain. Your child may have a problem if you notice, or they complain of, such symptoms as:

- Limping.
- Stiffness when awakening.
- Reluctance to use a limb.
- Reduced physical activity level.

Doctors will ask many questions about your child's symptoms. It is important to be open and honest with your doctor about all of the symptoms. One of the most important questions the doctor will ask is how long your child has shown symptoms. The swelling or pain must last for at least six weeks before the doctor will consider a juvenile rheumatoid arthritis diagnosis.

Physicians will also depend on a few diagnostic tests to help them determine if your child has arthritis, including:

- **Erythrocyte sedimentation rate (ESR):** This test measures how quickly red blood cells fall to the bottom of a test tube. Some people with rheumatic disease have an elevated level of red blood cells, which indicates inflammation in the body. Not all children with active joint inflammation will have an elevated ESR rate, however.

- **Rheumatoid factor:** a blood test to determine if your child has the RF factor, an abnormal antibody found in patients with rheumatoid arthritis. Children do not always have this factor, although they may have rheumatoid arthritis.

- **X-rays:** The doctor will order x-rays to make sure the joint pain or inflammation is not caused by an injury to the joint, or any unusual bone growth. X-rays are usually negative when a diagnosis of juvenile rheumatoid arthritis is made.

What causes juvenile rheumatoid arthritis?

Not all children will develop juvenile rheumatoid arthritis, so you are probably wondering why your child developed it and what caused it. There may have been certain risk factors that put your child at a higher risk for developing JRA, although pinpointing the exact cause may not always be possible.

Genetic predisposition

Researchers believe that rheumatoid arthritis may be triggered in people who have the "rheumatoid factor," known in the scientific literature as RA factor HLA-DR4. This appears to be a genetic marker on the surface of the cells. If a child is tested and found to have the rheumatoid factor, it means the child may have an inherited tendency toward developing rheumatoid arthritis and maintaining it throughout adulthood. Fewer than half of all the children with rheumatoid arthritis have the RF factor.

Viral infections

Some researchers believe that a viral infection triggers the rheumatoid arthritis in people who already possess the genetic marker for the disease. Since rheumatoid arthritis is an autoimmune disease, it is believed that the disease gets its start when the body's autoimmune system responds to a viral infection, and that once the infection has been successfully defeated, the autoimmune system does not stop its attack, but continues on to destroy the healthy cells.

Tumor Necrosis Factor (TNF)

Recently, another cause of rheumatoid arthritis has been uncovered. It is known as the tumor necrosis factor (TNF). TNF is a protein and chemical messenger, and it is an important part of the body's normal means to fight infections and injuries. During chronic illnesses, the body may overproduce TNF to harmful levels. In turn, these high levels of TNF can exacerbate the symptoms of a chronic illness, such as rheumatoid arthritis. Scientists are currently working on TNF blockers, or inhibitors, that can rein in the production of TNF before it causes any damage.

Low hormone levels

Researchers at the University of Iowa have shown a correlation between juvenile rheumatoid arthritis and low hormone levels in synovial fluid and serum

Bright Idea
Children with juvenile rheumatoid arthritis often have trouble brushing and flossing their teeth because joint pain prevents them from holding the toothbrush. Maintain regular visits to the dentist and inform your dentist of your child's health status, and consider buying an electric toothbrush, Water Pik and special rinses that may help your child keep his teeth clean.

AN IMPORTANT MESSAGE FROM THE USP

The United States Pharmacopeia (USP) has discovered that children—especially chronically ill children—are using medicines independently at very early ages. The USP states that one-third of all school children receive at least one prescription or over-the-counter drug every 48 hours. The more children know about medicines, the more prepared they are for responsible use as they get older. It is important for parents, guardians, and physicians to teach the children to:

- Take the right medicine at the right time in the right amount; read the directions with the child.

- Take all of the medicine prescribed even if he or she feels better. This is especially important when taking antibiotics.

- Report any unexpected side effects or reactions to an adult who can call a health care professional.

- Participate in health education activities that teach the principles of responsible medicine use.

- Tell an adult if the child thinks he has taken too much of a medicine so the local poison center can be notified as soon as possible.

Children usually get their medicine information from family, friends, and advertisements (in stores and publications, and on television). When asked, children say they want to learn about medicines from trusted sources such as their physician, teachers, or parents. As a parent, caregiver, or teacher, you can encourage children to ask their doctor about medicines and help them prepare appropriate questions. For example:

- What will my medicine taste like?
- How will it make me feel better?
- Will it be pills, liquids, or shots?
- When do I have to take it?
- How long to I have to take it?
- Does it have side effects?
- Why do I have to take it?

Treat medications seriously and store them out of reach and sight of young children.

Reprinted with permission by The U.S. Pharmacopeia (12601 Twinbrook Parkway, Rockville, MD 20852) e-mail: pjb@usp.org, 301-816-8118.

(the fluid portion of the blood). Researchers are still continuing with these studies to try to find out exactly how the low hormone levels trigger arthritis. Hopefully, this new research may lead to new preventatives and treatments.

Treatment

Unfortunately, there is no cure for juvenile rheumatoid arthritis, but there are medications to help dull the pain, reduce the stiffness and inflammation, and help to maintain normal joint function. How your child responds to treatment will vary from person to person, so it may take time to find the right combination.

Dulling the pain

Conventional therapy includes a combination of anti-inflammatory drugs and disease-modifying drugs that may slow the progression of the disease. Not all medications that have been approved for use in adults can be used with children. Here's a list of medications currently in use:

Nonsteroidal anti-inflammatory drugs (NSAIDs): The formal name for these medications is "nonsteroidal anti-inflammatory drugs"—commonly referred to as NSAIDs. Ibuprofen, naproxen sodium, Advil, Nuprin, Motrin, and Aleve are all NSAIDs. NSAIDs slow down the body's production of prostaglandins, substances that play a role in inflammation. They also carry some analgesic, or painkilling, properties as well. NSAIDs can be used if a patient does not respond to acetaminophen, but they must be carefully monitored for side effects. Side effects of these medications include gastrointestinal bleeding, kidney problems, dizziness, skin rash, and ringing in the ears.

To prevent some of the gastrointestinal irritation, it is recommended that NSAIDs should be taken with at least eight ounces of water. Do not lie down from 15 to 30 minutes after taking the drug to minimize irritation.

Arthrotec: If your child is at high risk for gastrointestinal complications caused by NSAIDs and aspirin, there may be relief in sight. Arthrotec, the brand name for diclofenac sodium, received U.S. marketing clearance from the Food and Drug Administration for patients who are at a high risk for complications caused by NSAIDs. Arthrotec consists of an enteric-coated core containing diclofenac sodium and misoprostol. There are side effects including abdominal pain, diarrhea, and stomach upset, but it is believed that these side effects are not as great as those caused by NSAIDs.

Watch Out!
Aspirin can cause Reye's syndrome in children who have or are recovering from a viral infection, such as chicken pox or influenza. Reye's syndrome is a very dangerous disease that can affect the brain and, in severe cases, may cause death.

Aspirin: Aspirin reduces fever, relieves pain, and reduces swelling and inflammation. It is one of the more popular forms of treatment because it is cheap and effective, but children are not usually given aspirin because it can cause stomach and intestinal problems, such as ulcers and bleeding. Using large doses of aspirin over a long period of time can also cause blood clotting defects and liver and kidney damage.

Acetaminophen: Acetaminophen is an aspirin-free pain reliever and fever reducer, as found in brands such as Tylenol. Acetaminophen is safe *when used as directed*, but side effects can include severe anemia.

Disease-modifying anti-rheumatic drugs: Disease-modifying anti-rheumatic drugs (DMARDs) work to slow or stop the basic progress of the disease. DMARDs may have to be taken for several weeks or months before any signs of improvement and are often combined with a NSAID. Some of the DMARDs include hydroxychloroquine, azulfidine, cyclosporine, sulfasalazine, azathioprine, d-pencillamine. The most frequently used DMARD for children is methotrexate.

Methotrexate has been used as an anti-cancer medicine, and is now a commonly used DMARD for rheumatoid arthritis. It is used, with supervision, in low doses to suppress the system enough to reduce swelling and slow down the damage and the progression of the disease. Methotrexate does have many side effects, including low white blood cell counts, gastrointestinal problems, sore throat, fever, nausea, and vomiting, but in low doses these side effects are rare.

Corticosteroids: Corticosteroids are synthetic versions of the hormone cortisone and include prednisone and dexamethasone. Corticosteroids are generally prescribed for short-term relief for an intense flare-up to immediately reduce pain and inflammation of severe juvenile rheumatoid arthritis and can be prescribed when patients do not find relief with other treatments. Unfortunately, while the relief is quick and dramatic, there can be serious side effects, including weight gain and thinning bones and skin. Corticosteroids can also interfere with the normal growth of a child and cause a rounded face, weakened bones, and susceptibility to infection. As a result, the use of corticosteroids is limited in children with juvenile arthritis. The shots are reserved for just a few times per year, or when absolutely necessary.

Physical therapy

It is important to help the child prevent or correct loss of range and function in the joints. Physical and occupational therapy can help preserve the mobility of the joint and strengthen the surrounding muscles and connective tissue. Your doctor may recommend splints and other devices. A regular exercise program is also recommended.

Surgery

Surgery on children with juvenile rheumatoid arthritis is only done as a last resort. The physician will exhaust every other treatment possibility before considering surgery. Surgery may be used to relieve pain, release joint contractures, or replace a damaged joint.

- **Joint contracture surgery:** Releasing joint contractures consists of cutting and repairing the tight tissue that caused the contracture, allowing the joint to return to a normal position.

- **Osteotomy:** The surgeon may suggest repositioning the joint, called an osteotomy. This surgical process consists of removing damaged bone and tissue and restoring the joint to its proper position. Recovery time from an osteotomy can be lengthy, perhaps from 6 to 12 months, and it does not guarantee that the function of the joint will improve. Additional treatment may be necessary. Whether or not your child will need another procedure, and when that procedure will take place, will depend on the condition of the joint before the procedure.

- **Synovectomy:** Synovectomy is a type of surgery in which the synovium, the membrane lining inside of a joint, is removed because it is inflamed and damaged by arthritis. Synovectomy is still performed, more commonly on fingers and knee joints.

- **Arthroplasty:** Arthroplasty, also called artificial joint replacement surgery, removes the diseased parts of the joint and replaces it with new, artificial parts made of metal and plastic. Although knees and hips are common joint replacements, there are over 2,000 wrist implants and 7,000 hand and finger implants inserted each year, according to *the Journal of the American Medical Association.* There are also artificial joints for shoulders, fingers, ankles, and wrists.

There are risks to every operation, and joint replacement surgery comes with its own set, including dislocation, inflammation, phlebitis (blood clots of a vein), damage to blood vessels and nerves, and possible revision surgery. If your physician has considered surgery for your child, discuss all the options and the risks involved.

How arthritis affects children

Having a chronic illness can affect a child emotionally, socially, and academically, not just physically. Emotionally, children may feel a wide variety of emotions, including anger and sadness that they are the ones that have to cope with daily pain. Children may feel as if they caused their own disease. They may feel different from their so-called "normal" friends—friends who do not have arthritis—and may feel resentful that they must eliminate or restrict certain activities because of their condition.

In severe cases, children with any form of arthritis may suffer from depression. It is important to know the symptoms of depression, to spot them in your child, and to get your child the necessary help. Symptoms of depression include:

Watch Out! Healthy siblings—especially very young ones—can easily come to resent the extra attention a sick child seems to receive. Be alert to signs of this happening in your household, and take steps to reassure the sibling(s) who feel left out that you love them just as much.

- Excessive crying.
- Anger.
- Isolation from other children.
- Restriction of activities.
- Change in school grades.
- Sleeping changes.
- Appetite changes.

How JRA affects the family

When you first heard that your child suffered from arthritis, you were probably shocked. Arthritis was probably the last medical condition that you would have guessed, right? After all, arthritis is popularly understood to be an "old person's disease." It is normal for parents to believe that they did something to cause the arthritis. It is also normal for them to feel guilty that they cannot do anything to repair it. One part of a parent's job is to kiss away their child's boo-boos, and when they find out that a boo-boo cannot just be kissed away, parents feel helpless. Parents also feel helpless when they watch their child in pain.

Get a caregiving schedule in place early

The demands on a family with a child that has a chronic illness can also be great. There may be many doctor appointments, medical tests, hospital and emergency room visits, surgeries, or therapy. This can result in a family schedule that often revolves around the needs of that child.

Some siblings of a child with a chronic illness are partial caregivers and are protective and proud of the accomplishments of that brother or sister. However, it is not uncommon for other siblings to feel isolated and jealous that the other child is getting so much attention. The siblings might not understand why.

Minimize sibling rivalry

There is tremendous pressure on the parents to make sure that all of their children are given the proper amount of attention, to prevent creating feelings of jealousy and isolation. There are important steps you can take to help your child and the family handle your child's illness.

- Treat the child who has arthritis as normally as possible. Do not give special privileges if the child is physically able to do something. Encourage normal physical and emotional development. Let the child participate in regular school activities, extracurricular activities, and family responsibilities.

- Talk to *all* of your children and allow each of them, healthy and ill, the chance to express feelings of anger or frustration.

- Encourage your children to find, and employ, their own special talents.

- Encourage the child with arthritis, and his siblings, to learn as much as possible about the disease.

- As your child gets older, prepare her for living independently with arthritis.

- Talk with teachers and school administrators about your child's arthritis and work with them to find the best way to prepare your child and for the school to handle the condition.

- Consider joining a support group that will put you in touch with other people in your own (and your child's) situation.

Moneysaver
Numerous doctor and prescription bills can put a dent in anyone's budget. Supplemental Security Income (SSI) is a monthly payment from the Social Security Administration to people of any age who are disabled if they have limited income and resources. In many states, children who receive SSI automatically qualify for Medicaid. Contact the Social Security Administration at (800) 722-1213.

That last item is key for many people. The American Juvenile Arthritis Organization runs support groups for people with JRA and their families. A support group is a group of people with a common condition that meet on a regular basis to share stories, advice, and emotional support. Support groups can also be a forum in which you can learn practical information about your child's condition, such as the most recent medical information, or the latest diagnostic technology. This is also a good opportunity for your child to meet other children in the area who are afflicted with arthritis. For parents and caregivers, it is an opportunity to exchange tips and advice on caring for children with arthritis.

You may be eligible for additional resources, such as assistance through state agencies or vocational rehabilitation. Contacting other families who are dealing with similar issues may be helpful, and the American Juvenile Arthritis Organization provides educational material, conferences, and networking opportunities.

Looking ahead

Researchers are still investigating the causes of juvenile rheumatoid arthritis, in particular, the genetic and environmental factors of the disease. The NIAMSD has established a research registry for families in which two or more siblings have juvenile rheumatoid arthritis. The organization also funds a Multipurpose Arthritis and Musculoskeletal Diseases Center that specializes in pediatric rheumatic diseases and research. To get more information about the Research Registry contact:

Edward Giannini, MD
Children's Hospital Medical Center–PAV 2-129
University of Cincinnati, College of Medicine
Cincinnati, OH 45229
(513) 636-7634 or (513) 636-4495
E-mail: btague@one.net
or visit their web site at: http://www.jraregistry.org.

For more information about the MAMDC, contact:
David Glass, MD
Children's Hospital Medical Center–PAV 2-129
University of Cincinnati, College of Medicine
Cincinnati, OH 45229
(513) 636-8854
E-mail: glasd0@chmcc.org
or visit their web site at: http://www.cinciMAMDC.org

Just the facts

- Juvenile rheumatoid arthritis affects more than 70,000 children; most of them are girls.

- Children with JRA can suffer from depression; learn how to spot the symptoms early.

- Children with JRA do not need to minimize or restrict their activities, unless it hurts them.

- It is important for the entire family, not just the child who has arthritis to learn as much as they can about the condition. Arthritis affects the entire family.

Treatment and Medication

GET THE SCOOP ON...
Snake oil remedies ▪ Folk treatments ▪
Supplements ▪ Experimental therapies ▪
Spotting a quack

PART III

Chapter 8

Deciphering Truth from Quackery

Coping with the aches and pains of arthritis is a daily struggle. On some days, you may find that you are able to manage the discomfort, inflammation, and lack of mobility. On other days, just making it through breakfast may seem overwhelming. You may feel so desperate for a cure that you will try anything. Then, as if it were fate, staring up at you from your morning newspaper is an advertisement for a miracle cure.

The problem for arthritis sufferers is this: How do you distinguish between the hype and the helpful? After all, *some* truly useful therapies do come from outside of mainstream medicine.

In this chapter you'll learn about all the magical miracle cures being pitched to arthritis sufferers, and you'll get the lowdown on product claims and hype—and how to spot the useful alternatives among the fakes.

Looking for hope wherever you can find it

Advertisements for miracle arthritis cures typically claim that you can eliminate your pain in days. They urge you to read the persuasive testimonials from previous users, which are attributed to arthritis sufferers who describe symptoms that are similar to yours, and report how they are now free from pain, thanks to this special, magical cure. You feel that they must understand your plight of suffering.

The offer to be cured from your arthritis sounds so good, and all you have to do is simply mail a check to receive your first shipment of a "cure-all" medication, or miraculous device, that will just melt your arthritic pains away. Your joints ache, desperation sets in, and you mail your check immediately.

Caveat emptor—let the buyer beware!

Unfortunately, you may have just put your health at risk. These self-proclaimed cure-alls are anything but, and many of these products that allege to be breakthroughs in treating or eliminating arthritis are unproven, and possibly dangerous, remedies. If you have already fallen for one of these deceptive cures, do not feel foolish. Many smart, educated consumers are lured into buying these products because of suggestive wording and promises of cures.

The U.S. Food and Drug Administration (FDA) estimates that 38 million Americans have used a fraudulent health product within the past year and, according to Medical World News, spent about $27 billion a year on quack products or treatments.

As of yet, no matter what companies may headline in their advertisements, there are no medically-proven cures for arthritis, only relief for

Unofficially... Yankees pitcher Hidecki Irabu wears small circular magnetic pressure bandages when he pitches. The Museum of Questionable Medical Devices reports that these bandages were sold in the 1970s as a cure for minor aches and pains. The magnets were said to attract iron in the blood and increase circulation. One small problem: Iron is a mineral, not a metal, and would not be attracted to the magnets.

symptoms. So-called miracle cures are far more likely to:

- Waste your money.
- Cost you time from getting early, professional treatment.
- Cause side effects.
- Endanger your life.

There are proven treatments that can help alleviate your symptoms, but your health is in your own hands. Do not just try anything to ease the pain. Learn fact from fiction when it comes to treating your body. This chapter will give you the confidence to make the right consumer decisions that protect both your wallet and your health.

Snake oil salespeople

According to the U.S. Food and Drug Administration's 1996 list of Top Health Frauds in the United States, fraudulent arthritis products are number one. While it is possible for some people to feel better with the use of these products, the FDA illustrates that arthritis is a condition that can go into remission and flare-up again, later. During remission, individuals may associate the improvement in their health with the remedy that they have tried. In turn, the manufacturers of these products have created a false sense of hope in the patients. The patients then continue to buy more and more of the product.

Today, health care fraud is a billion-dollar industry. Promoters, quacks, or snake oil salespeople, claim that their skills or products have curative powers, and they prey on innocent victims who suffer from such ailments that have no cure, such as arthritis.

Watch Out!
If you are currently taking any medications for your arthritis, consult your physician and pharmacist before you start using a new unproven treatment. Mixing prescribed medications with a natural home-made remedy or supplement can cause side effects, or death. Better to be safe than sorry.

You might think that in the age of modern medicine, individuals or companies would have been stopped from selling fraudulent products. Unfortunately, fraudulent products are still being marketed and sold.

Who buys these products?

Everyone is vulnerable, regardless of education level, to being taken in by a fraudulent claim. According to the Mayo Clinic, people who purchase fraudulent products often have similar characteristics, including:

- They tend to be isolated, lacking the emotional support of family and friends.

- Their illness has lead to a sense of "losing control over their lives."

- They may have chronic or incurable diseases.

- They may have problems that can also cause emotional distress, such as impotence, baldness, and excess weight.

People who manufacture quackery products thrive on the vulnerability of the sick. Your desperation for a cure may have turned you into an unsuspecting victim of a quackery product, and you do not realize it until after the fact.

The first step in avoiding quackery products is to become educated about the various products that are on the market and how to spot the questionable treatments.

Moneysaver
If you wish to report a suspected quackery, or snake-oil, sales pitch, call the National Fraud Information Center at 1-800-876-7060.

Folk remedies

Folk, or traditional medicine, consists of typically homemade remedies, sometimes herbal in nature, and often based on superstition. Some have been shown to be helpful in easing arthritis pain, some have not. All share the characteristic of being derived from folk, rather than Western scientific, tradition.

Apple cider vinegar and honey is one example of a folk remedy that has been extolled as a solution for just about everything over the years, including arthritis pain. Author and physician D.C. Jarvis wrote a popular book about its benefits and use by Vermont residents, but apple cider vinegar and honey remains an unproven remedy.

Hundreds of other folk remedies have claimed to cure arthritis or eliminate the pain. In the following sections we'll discuss just a few.

Capsicum peppers

Capsicum is the "pepper" in the self-defense weapon pepper-spray. It contains capsaicin, a very pungent phenolic chemical, and produces a feeling of warmth throughout the body. Once it is ingested, you will begin to sweat and your eyes and nose will begin to water. Capsaicin is now a salve that has been approved by the FDA for pain relief and is sold under various brand names. It does not cure arthritis, but can help to relieve pain.

Cayenne pepper

Cayenne pepper has a rich history in folk medicine—and some companies are bottling it and marketing it as a panacea, or cure-all, for most diseases or illnesses. Cayenne pepper follows the same physiological response as capsicum peppers, but its effectiveness has not been studied. However, it has shown some usefulness in treating arthritis pain.

Snake venom

Using snake venom to cure an illness may sound horrifying, but some believe that it works. Although

Unofficially...
Samuel Thomson, leader of the antiphysician movement of the early 1800s, was a strong believer in the use of cayenne pepper.

Unofficially...
Keeping track of what's helpful and what's hype is tricky. One thing to remember is that FDA approval is not the only criterion to go by. All that approval really means is that the substance has been tested in a laboratory—but many folk remedies aren't tested, even if they've been used effectively.

it has not been medically proven as a cure for arthritis, researchers at the University of Southern California are now researching snake venom's ability to cure cancer. Researchers have isolated a protein from snake toxins and are testing its effectiveness in stopping the spread of cancer cells throughout the body. However, snake venom has not been proven to be a cure or treatment for arthritis. The result can be fatal if you attempt to self-medicate.

Bee venom

Like snake venom, bee venom is alleged to have properties that can reduce the inflammation in the arthritic joint and reduce the aches and pains. Patients who use bee venom subject themselves to painful bee stings. The treatment is repeated on the infected area, and over a period of time, it is believed that the patient develops an immunity to the stings. Once this happens, the patient reportedly receives the maximum benefit from the venom.

There have been many animal studies on the use of bee venom, but while these studies have had some positive outcomes, the medical community has not embraced the theory yet that bee venom can help to relieve suffering.

Dental fillings and arthritis

Every week for years, millions of viewers have tuned into 60 Minutes on Sunday nights. This hour-long show made a dramatic impact on the informative value of television. However, on December 23, 1990, reporter Morley Safer narrated a segment on mercury amalgam dental fillings. This segment claimed the fillings are toxic and can be contributing to various diseases and disorders of your body, including arthritis. By removing the fillings, you would balance your body and eliminate these illnesses.

This has to be one of the most controversial segments in the 60 Minutes broadcast history. The report sparked a nationwide scare that rivaled the famed Orson Wells "War of the Worlds" broadcast.

An article in Consumer Reports magazine says, "My mother…had her mercury fillings removed immediately after the show aired. After she had spent $10,000 and endured more than 18 hours of dental work so painful she once fainted in the waiting room, her condition did not improve. The pain was outweighed only by the monumental disappointment she and the whole family experienced as we lived through one false hope."

Do not rush to the dentist just yet to have all your fillings removed. Although this show triggered fear in arthritis sufferers and many people do believe in the so-called harmful fillings, amalgam fillings have not been proven to be harmful.

Chuifong toukuwan

According to the Food and Drug Administration, Chuifong toukuwan is a Chinese herbal medication that was promoted as an arthritis cure in the late 1970s. Unfortunately, in 1980, several illnesses and deaths were linked to use of this medication.

The FDA also reported that in 1983, an additional brand of Chuifong toukuwan variety labeled only in Chinese appeared in the Portland, Oregon area. In 1988, the Food and Drug Branch of the California State Department of Health Services announced an enforcement initiative against dangerous Chinese and other Asian ethnic medicines. These products are currently off the market and have not been proven to be safe or effective.

Unofficially...
According to *Bee Culture* magazine, Hippocrates has been known to use bee stings in his ministrations, Galen (AD 130) wrote of bee venom treatment, and Charlemagne was purported to have received bee stings as treatment for stiff joints.

Copper bracelets

Some folk remedies, like snake venom or Chuifong toukuwan, are potentially fatal if used incorrectly. Some folk remedies, such as copper bracelets, are harmless.

Who knows where the first claims that copper heals arthritis came from? Whatever the source of these claims, lots of people believe that wearing copper close to your skin helps arthritis sufferers. The belief is that the copper, absorbed through your skin, neutralizes the "bad guys"—the free radicals—in your body. This is supposed to eliminate your pain.

Unfortunately, there's no scientific evidence whatsoever to support these claims. And while you may indeed absorb trace amounts of copper from your bracelet, it has no discernible effect on the free radicals. While there's little likelihood of copper having any effect on your arthritis, it is, at least, harmless.

Apple cider vinegar and honey

In 1992, one company manufactured a new mixture of grape and apple juices and vinegar and claimed that, with honey, its benefits included eliminating arthritis and heart disease, and reducing the risk of cancer in the internal organs. These claims were unsubstantiated and the product was removed from the market and destroyed.

Presently, due to the high potassium level in vinegar, an apple cider vinegar mixture has been recommended as a homeopathic, natural solution for leg cramps, but there is no medical evidence definitely linking apple cider vinegar and honey to eliminating arthritis pain.

Supplements

Supplements are widely available in health food and drug stores, but consumers are warned that the FDA does not regulate these products unless serious harm from their use is demonstrated. Make sure you tell your doctor if you are taking supplements, what types, and how much. If you notice any adverse effects from taking any of these products, notify FDA MedWatch, 5600 Fishers Ln, Rockville, MD 20852-9787; (800) FDA-0178.

Glucosamine sulfate and chondroitin exploded onto the health food store shelves a few years ago when one book touted the supplement as the hottest remedy for osteoarthritis sufferers. The book claimed that the wear and tear of the joint that causes osteoarthritis is due to excess action of enzymes that break down cartilaginous tissue in the normal maintenance of joints. The author claimed that the glucosamine sulfate and chondroitin supplements help to replace this tissue.

Glucosamine is found in high concentrations in the joints. Scientists are currently studying the effect glucosamine may have in slowing down the cartilage breakdown, relieving pain, and increasing your range of motion.

There have been some promising studies linking glucosamine and osteoarthritis. However, the American College of Rheumatology has informed consumers that these early animal studies and short-term human studies are not 100 percent convincing, and additional studies are still needed to confirm these results.

The FDA position on supplements

The FDA states that a manufacturer cannot claim that their product can *cure* any disease until it has undergone rigorous testing and the FDA issues its approval. The FDA will not consider authorizing the manufacturer to promote any health claim unless there is significant scientific proof that the claim is valid.

Unfortunately, this FDA requirement does not guarantee that manufacturers will comply with the law. There are many unauthorized claims on products that have not been removed.

Contraptions and gadgets

Quackery products are not limited to supplements. For thousands of years, individuals have been inventing gadgets—such as electrical stimulators, vibrating objects, and peculiar-looking devices that look more like a child's toy than a medical device— in an attempt to cure arthritis or to eliminate the pain and aches.

These companies claim that their products are adequate and effective treatments for various forms of arthritis. Some products claim to electrically stimulate cartilage and joints, or heat the arthritic area and thereby decrease the pain. Some products are harmless, but some can incorrectly stimulate the afflicted area and actually cause additional pain. As a result, you may have more medical problems than you began with.

One such device was the Stimulator, a device that looks like an electric gas barbecue grill igniter with fingertips. The manufacturers of this device claimed that the Stimulator relieved many ailments, including arthritis. However, the company did not comply with FDA regulations that govern the marketing and sale of medical devices, and the product has been investigated and removed.

Unofficially...
One of the earliest medical gadgets was devised in 1770 by American Elisha Perkins. The "Perkins Tractors" were metal rods, which were intended to cure nervous ailments and other ailments, including arthritis. George Washington was known to have used this product.

Unproven or experimental?

Two words that manufacturers use when introducing new products to consumers are "unproven" and "experimental." While they may sound the same, there is a big difference between the two.

The folk remedies and gadgets that have already been discussed are unproven, which means that they have not been subjected to scientific testing or, if they have, the results have been inconclusive. However, if the treatments are in an experimental stage of testing, then the product is currently undergoing testing, but the tests are not yet complete.

How experimental drugs are developed

The experimental stage may take years to complete. In 1996, researchers at the Thomas Jefferson University claimed to have developed an experimental vaccine that seemed to subdue the symptoms of rheumatoid arthritis. The researchers called the initial findings "promising," and additional testing is still being completed. We may not hear about this "promising" vaccine for another 10 or 20 years. Other examples of treatments in the experimental stage include:

- Gene therapy.
- Powdered shark cartilage.

The cutting-edge research of gene therapy

What is a gene? When a baby is conceived, a mother's ovum, or egg, is joined by a father's sperm and an embryo is formed. The egg and the sperm each contain 23 chromosomes, for a total of 46 when they are joined together. Inside these chromosomes are genes, or little pockets of information, that determine your characteristics, from whether or not you were a boy or girl, to your hair and eye color, and your height. It also includes information on diseases that can be inherited or passed from your parents to you. Normal, healthy genes can also be damaged from environmental causes that may trigger potential diseases.

One of the most remarkable discoveries this century is that scientists have identified specific genes that cause various illnesses, such as lupus, rheumatoid arthritis, and scleroderma. For example, the discovery of the "rheumatoid factor," or the genetic factor that may cause rheumatoid arthritis, was an important advance for arthritis sufferers.

Recently scientists have also found a way to isolate some of these faulty genes and repair or eliminate them. As a result, there is a chance that a disease, such as rheumatoid arthritis, can be stamped out of your body.

The first experiment with gene therapy for rheumatoid arthritis was conducted on a 68-year-old woman. Doctors removed cells from her thumb joint, reproduced them in a laboratory, then modified them to carry a gene that blocks inflammation. Analysis is currently being done to determine if the gene therapy was successful.

In the meantime, since the gene has been identified, genetic screening tests can determine if you have the gene that carries a disease. The testing only requires a simple blood sample.

The Arthritis Foundation, the National Institute of Arthritis, Musculoskeletal and Skin Diseases (NIAMSD) and the National Institute of Allergy and Infectious Diseases (NIAID) are collaborating on a national consortium of ten research centers in search for more genes that will help to determine any susceptibility to rheumatoid arthritis.

This study, known as the North American Rheumatoid Arthritis Consortium (NARAC), will take three to five years to complete. The goal of the NARAC is to collect medical information and genetic material (DNA) from 1,000 families nationwide. These families should have two or more siblings who developed rheumatoid arthritis when they were between 18 and 60 years of age and have at least one surviving parent. For more information, or to inquire about participating in the study, you can contact NARAC at (800) 382-4827, or visit their web site at http://medicine.ucsf.edu.

Powdered shark cartilage

Sharks have no bones; their skeletal structure is all cartilage. Human cartilage is a rubbery substance that protects the bone and reduces the friction between two bones.

Shark cartilage is rich in calcium and phosphorus and contains chondroitin sulfate, an anti-inflammatory agent. Researchers believe that sharks are naturally disease-free, and that lack of disease may be linked to their cartilage. However, although studies have offered some hope that shark cartilage may have some beneficial components for humans, more research is necessary before it is proven to be an effective treatment for arthritis pain.

Hemicallotasis

Hemicallotasis is a funny name for a strange treatment, but doctors at Temple University Hospital in Philadelphia claim it works.

To eliminate pain caused by arthritic knees, surgeons at Temple University intentionally fracture the knees of patients on the side where the cartilage has worn away. Then the surgeons insert screws into the bone on either side of the fracture and connect

Watch Out!
Remember,
there's a differ-
ence between
the words
"proven" and
"approved." A
product may
have demon-
strated effective-
ness but not
have been
tested.

them with a rod. The patient then turns a dial on the rod once a day, which expands the bone and pulls apart the fracture one millimeter a day. As the fracture widens, new bone grows in the crack and fills it in.

The purpose is to shift a patient's weight off of the area in the knee where the cartilage has worn away. Arthritic knees are caused by the wearing away of cartilage between bone, causing the bones of a joint to rub against each other. If the cartilage has worn away on the part of the knee that bears the brunt of a person's weight, the pain is even worse. According to surgeons, hemicallotasis can eliminate joint pain by shifting the weight of the person to the other side of the knee.

This procedure is currently being performed on younger arthritic patients. Although it is relatively new in the medical community, its long-term effects are still unknown.

Keep in mind that there are many medications and procedures that started out as experimental, but after successfully completing scientific trials, have gone on to become accepted as effective treatments. Methotrexate, for example, was once considered an experimental treatment for arthritis. Now it is an FDA-approved medication prescribed for rheumatoid arthritis patients who do not respond to standard treatment.

Unproven treatments

If a product has been scientifically tested, there is still no guarantee that the product is effective. An unproven treatment means that the treatment or product has either failed to undergo scientific testing, or has not shown any conclusive evidence that it works or does what it claims to do. It is risky to use an unproven medical treatment. Without knowing the side effects, you are putting your health at risk. Some unproven treatments are dangerous and can even be fatal if used incorrectly.

Some of these dangerous, unproven remedies include:

Dimethyl sulfoxide
Dimethyl sulfoxide is a solvent that is similar to turpentine, a cleaning fluid, and has been promoted for arthritis relief. It is one of the few compounds that the skin absorbs rapidly, but there are no medical studies that demonstrate its safety and effectiveness in relieving swollen, inflamed arthritic joints. It can also be potentially dangerous if it is used as an enema, as directed by the manufacturer.

Dimethyl sulfoxide is, however, an FDA-approved medication for treating a rare bladder condition called interstitial cystitis.

Germanium
This is a non-essential element sold as a dietary supplement. Manufacturers claim that applying bandage-wraps saturated with germanium can reduce the pain and inflammation of arthritic joints. While it has not yet been FDA approved, it enjoys a good reputation among holistic health practitioners.

Gerovital-H3
This product was brought to the United States illegally from Romania more than 30 years ago. One of the ingredients in Gerovital-H3 is procaine hydrochloride, an anesthetic approved for dental use. Manufacturers sold it as a cure for arthritis and other conditions, and it has a long history of use in holistic medicine.

Misinformation superhighway

You probably obtain your medical information from many different sources including:

- Physicians.
- Friends and family.
- Medical reference books.
- Newspaper magazines and articles.

Over the past few years, many have turned to the Internet as a source of medical information. The Internet has become one of our most important and commonly used research tools. However, just because the Internet provides a wealth of medical information does not make it the most accurate or reliable source of information.

In November 1997, the Federal Trade Commission reported that more than 400 web sites and numerous Usenet newsgroups contained promotions for products and services claiming to cure, treat, or prevent many illnesses, including arthritis. In what was called North American Health Claims Surf Day, the FTC sent hundreds of e-mail messages to web sites and newsgroups pointing out that advertisers must have evidence to support their claims.

This alarming number of fraudulent web sites should encourage all consumers to be on guard for deceptive products.

Spotting a quack

Are you confident that you could spot a quack doctor, treatment, or medication? Even the most educated consumers can be lured into buying false products through enticing advertisements and promises of cures.

How can you spot a deceptive product? Look to see if the packaging or advertisements make claims such as these:

- The product "cures everything" from aches and pains, to acne, dandruff, and more serious diseases, such as arthritis and cancer. No one product can do all of these things.

- The manufacturer of the product promises a "quick and easy cure." But you've got to ask yourself: What does easy mean?

- The product is described as "harmless" or "natural."

Unsubstantiated claims like these are against the law. Other key words to look for include:

- Exclusive.

- Secret.

- Miraculous.

Now let's return to our original advertisement that sparked your interest and prompted you to send in money hoping for a cure. The advertisement illustrated how you could eliminate your arthritis pain in days. The advertisement urged you to read the persuasive testimonials from previous users. The testimonials described symptoms that are similar to yours, and how these patients are now free from pain. You felt that they must understand your plight of suffering. But, before you send in any money, consider the following:

- *The manufacturers claim that the medical community does not accept the product.* Any manufacturer who discovers a cure for any disease or condition will definitely be taken seriously by the medical community. In most cases, this claim means that the item may have been tested, but not proven to be successful.

When the pitchman makes conspiratorial claims, such as "based on a secret formula" or

"Dr. X just invented a new product that will eliminate arthritis pain," watch out. Such claims are frequently followed up with the charge that "the medical community does not want to acknowledge this top secret product." According to the FDA, however, legitimate scientists who have researched and proven their product with proper medical studies will share their knowledge so that their peers can review the data. Once a treatment is proven effective, practitioners in the medical community are free to use it.

Moneysaver
For a free FTC brochure called "Fraudulent Health Claims: Don't be fooled," call 202-326-2222 or visit the FTC web site at www.ftc.gov. If you have problems with a company that you believe is selling fraudulent products, contact the local Better Business Bureau, Attorney General's Office, or Postmaster if you purchased the product by mail.

■ *The product only cites one study.* One study is not enough to claim a breakthrough on any medication or treatment. More studies must be done to confirm the initial findings. Therefore, if a manufacturer claims all of the benefits of the medication or treatment from the one study, wait and see what other studies are done and if they agree with the first study. If the product is a true cure, the results will repeat themselves.

The Federal Trade Commission (FTC) requires a claim for any over-the-counter drug to be supported by two adequate and well-controlled studies, or handled in accordance with claims approved by the FDA for the product. According to the FTC, an adequate and well-controlled study is one done by independent investigators, where the tested ingredient is compared to a control (either another active ingredient or a placebo, or mock drug) and where the medications compared are not known to patients or investigators.

■ *The study cited has only been published in obscure publication, not in respected medical journals.* Even if the advertisement cites several studies, check to see if they've been documented in reputable medical journals. Any product that has been scientifically tested will be reported in refereed journals, such as the Journal of the American Medical Association or the New England Journal of Medicine, not just advertised on mail-order pages or in infomercials.

Getting the product

Okay, so you did go and order the treatment or product. Once you receive the package, take a close look at its contents for these:

- Is it packaged poorly?
- Does the product come with directions?
- Does the packaging list the product contents?
- Does the packaging include information or warnings about the side effects from using the product?
- Is there a way to contact the manufacturer in case you have side effects?

Consumers who have questions or wish to report a company for falsely labeling its products should contact the FDA's Office of Consumer Affairs at 5600 Fishers Lane, HFC-110, Rockville, MD 20857; or call (304) 443-3170. Or contact the Federal Trade Commission, Sixth and Pennsylvania Avenues, NW, Washington, DC 20580. If the product was delivered through the mail, contact the U.S. Postal Service Chief Postal Inspector, 475 L'Enfant Plaza, Washington, DC 20260.

Finding the quack

Snake oil salesmen are not always caught after claims of fraud are made against them. When these

Bright Idea
The National Council Against Health Fraud at Consumers urge consumers who have suffered from a serious adverse reaction associated with the use of a dietary supplement to their health care professional or to MedWatch at (800) FDA-1088.

slick salespersons feel that the heat is on they may either move from state to state or change their business name.

If you believe you have been sold a fraudulent product, contact the National Council Against Health Fraud. This organization can refer you to a lawyer. Contact them at (909) 824-4690.

Sometimes people do get better while using unproven treatments or remedies. But do not automatically assume that your symptoms improve because of the treatment. Your disease may have gone into remission, or there may be additional factors involved in your success.

Just the facts

- Don't be quick to spend your money for a new treatment or device that claims to help your arthritis. Conduct your own research on the product.

- Not all devices or unproven treatments are dangerous or useless, but it is important to become an educated consumer to learn the difference.

- Notify your physician of anything you try to help reduce your pain. Keep a notebook to track treatments, dates, methods, etc.

- If you have tried an unproven remedy and are suffering from side effects, let your physician know immediately.

GET THE SCOOP ON...
First- and second-line medications ▪
Protecting your stomach ▪ Deadly results:
combining medications

Chapter 9

Medications:
Temporary Relief

The sad truth is this: There are, at present, no medical cures for arthritis pain and inflammation. The medications that your physician prescribes for your symptoms can merely provide temporary relief for your symptoms.

This chapter will examine the choices available to you and provide you with a basic understanding of the terminology, descriptions, and side effects of the medications you are taking. New medications are introduced frequently, as are changes to dosages or reports of new side effects. Because the field of arthritis pain relief medication is changing so rapidly, this chapter cannot be exhaustive—make sure you speak with your physician about any questions you may have about your medications.

From aspirin to necrosis factor blockers: a brief history of pain relief

Today, physicians have a wide variety of medications to choose from and prescribe to help alleviate your

173

symptoms. Only a few decades ago, arthritis sufferers depended almost solely on aspirin to reduce the pain and inflammation. Then products containing acetaminophen, such as Tylenol, became available, giving arthritis sufferers an alternative that would not affect their stomachs by causing gastrointestinal distress as much aspirin did.

Through the years, the list of medications available to patients with arthritis has continued to grow, and researchers are developing more medications every day. In the past two years alone, patients who suffer from rheumatoid arthritis and osteoarthritis have been introduced to many new medications. Leflunomide, also known by its brand name, Arava, was the first of the "second-line medications" introduced in the last ten years for rheumatoid arthritis sufferers (second-line medications are discussed in greater detail later in this chapter). Synvisc and Hyalgan, known generically as sodium hyaluronate, are two other new medications developed for osteoarthritis sufferers. Sodium hyaluronate is injected into the affected site to prevent irritation. Enbrel is the first tumor necrosis factor blocker that has been approved by the Food and Drug Administration. Arthritis sufferers have also seen the introduction of Arthrotec, Celebrex—the first Cox-2 inhibitor approved by the FDA for treatment. Both of these medications will help reduce your risk of side effects from taking NSAIDs.

When deciding on your pain-management strategy, however, the most important thing to remember is *not* the number of medicinal choices. The most important thing to remember is to take your medications properly, according to your physician's orders, and to notify your physician of any potential complications or side effects from your medications. It is also important to take your medications responsibly: Do not consume alcohol, or share your medications with others. This might sound like obvious advice, but when you, or your friends or relatives, are in so much pain from arthritis, it is possible for desperation to set in. This leads to mistakes in judgement, which could be damaging to your body.

First-line medications

First-line medications are just that—the first medications that doctors will prescribe to relieve joint inflammation and pain. There are several options in this category of drugs:

Acetaminophen

Acetaminophen is an aspirin-free pain reliever and fever reducer, such as Tylenol. Acetaminophen is safe when used as directed, but side effects can include severe anemia.

Nonsteroidal anti-inflammatory drugs

Also known as NSAIDs, these first-line medications slow down the body's production of prostaglandins, substances that play a role in inflammation. NSAIDs also carry some analgesic, or pain-killing, properties. Aspirin, ibuprofen, and naproxen are just some examples of NSAIDs. Brand name, over-the-counter versions of NSAIDs include Advil, Nuprin, Motrin, and Aleve. NSAIDs are usually prescribed if you do not respond to acetaminophen, but you must be carefully monitored for any potential side effects, including:

gastrointestinal irritation

ulcers

dizziness

skin rashes

ringing in the ears

abdominal burning

pain

cramping

nausea

gastrointestinal bleeding

To reduce your risk of some of the side effects of NSAIDs, it is recommended that you:

- Take NSAIDs with at least eight ounces of water.

- Take NSAIDs with food (check with your physician and pharmacist).

- Do not lie down for at least 15 to 30 minutes after taking the medication.

- Take an antacid with the medication, such as TUMS. An antacid will act as a buffer and absorb the acid created by the NSAID in your stomach.

- Stay out of the sun, as NSAIDs can increase your sensitivity to it. To accomplish this, stay out of direct sunlight, especially between 10 a.m. and 3 p.m., wear protective clothing, and apply a sunblock for extra protection.

It is not unusual for your physician to try several NSAIDs in order to determine which medication provides the most effectiveness with the fewest side effects.

Aspirin

Aspirin is one of the most popular forms of pain relievers, because it is cheap and effective. Aspirin relieves pain and reduces fever, swelling, and inflammation.

Unofficially...
The Centers for Disease Control and Prevention in Atlanta estimate that NSAID related complications lead to 76,000 hospitalizations and 7,600 deaths each year.

Like other NSAIDs, it can also cause stomach and intestinal problems, such as ulcers and bleeding. Consuming large doses of aspirin over a long period of time can also cause blood clotting problems and damage to the liver and kidneys.

If you want to take aspirin, take an aspirin that has an enteric coating. An enteric coating means that the aspirin will not release its contents until it reaches your intestines, thereby eliminating the stomach irritation. However, it may take longer for you to obtain pain relief. In some cases, aspirin may be prescribed at very high doses. If so, you must be closely monitored for side effects.

Watch Out!
Patients with a history of asthma attacks, hives, or other allergic reactions to aspirin should avoid NSAIDs.

Corticosteroids

Corticosteroids are synthetic versions of the hormone cortisone and include prednisone, dexamethasone, and hydrocortisone. There are several benefits to corticosteroids for reducing inflammation:

1. Corticosteroid medications can be given orally or injected directly into tissues and joints.

2. Corticosteroids are more potent than NSAIDs in reducing inflammation, and in restoring joint mobility and function.

3. Corticosteroids are useful for short periods during severe flares of disease activity, and when the inflammation is not responding to NSAIDs.

However, corticosteroids can have serious side effects, especially when given in high doses for long periods of time. These side effects include:

- Weight gain.
- Facial puffiness.
- Thinning of the skin and bones.
- Easy bruising.

- Cataracts.

- Risk of infection.

- Destruction of large joints, such as the hips.

Do not abruptly stop taking corticosteroids. This can lead to a flare-up of your symptoms. Instead there should be a gradual weaning of corticosteroids.

The second-line

While first-line medications are prescribed to help relieve joint inflammation and pain, these medications do not necessarily prevent the arthritis from destroying the joint. To slow down the progression of the disease, "second-line" or "slow-acting" medicines can be prescribed. Second-line medications are also called "disease-modifying anti-rheumatic drugs" (DMARDs) or "immunosuppressive drugs" because they modify or suppress the disease.

Second-line medications include, but are not limited to, methotrexate, azathioprine, cyclophosphamide, chlorambucil, cyclosporin, azulfidine, sulfasalazine, and d-pencillamine. This class of medication must be used for long periods of time, and it may take months before you notice any benefits from the medications. Physicians may prescribe second-line medications with first-line medications as a combination therapy to help slow down the symptoms and reduce pain and inflammation at the same time.

Second-line medicines can cause serious side effects, and are generally reserved for patients with very severe arthritis, or those with serious complications of rheumatoid inflammation. Side effects include:

Bright Idea
Studies have shown that patients who must take a medication regularly will only take it correctly 50 to 75 percent of the time. You will not gain the benefits of your medications if you do not take them correctly. Use a pillbox, calendar, or timer to remind you to take your medication.

- Liver disease.
- Fertility difficulties.
- Birth defects.
- Spontaneous abortion.
- Mouth sores.
- Gastrointestinal irritations.
- Sore throat.
- Fever.
- Nausea.
- Vomiting.
- Allergic lung reactions.

Methotrexate

This is probably the most commonly prescribed DMARD for arthritis. Methotrexate is used to treat psoriasis, an inflammatory skin disease, as well as psoriatic arthritis. It is also used to treat rheumatoid arthritis.

Penicillamine

Penicillamine is used to treat active rheumatoid arthritis and scleroderma. Patients who take penicillamine should not take gold treatments.

Azathioprine

The exact benefit of azathioprine as a treatment for rheumatoid arthritis is not yet known, but it does have an effect in suppressing the immune system.

Gold salts

Gold treatments have been used for years to treat arthritis. Gold salts, which contain real gold as a dissolved salt, can be given orally or injected directly into the affected site. Gold salts, like other DMARDs, need to be used for an extended period

Watch Out!
Methotrexate can cause serious liver disease, so patients with alcoholism or liver diseases should not take it. Limit your alcohol intake while on this drug.

of time to gain the maximum benefits. Studies have also shown that you might gain similar benefits of gold salts by wearing gold rings. Gold rings may actually delay the progression of rheumatoid arthritis in the fingers on which they are worn.

There are minor side effects to using gold salts, including:

- Skin rashes.
- Mouth ulcers.
- Itching.
- Dizziness.
- Fainting.

Patients receiving gold salt treatments are regularly monitored with blood and urine tests.

Leflunomide

Leflunomide, also known by its brand name, Arava, is the first DMARD approved specifically to treat rheumatoid arthritis to be made available in more than 10 years. Leflunomide blocks the overproduction of immune cells that are responsible for most of the inflammation. Leflunomide has been shown to have positive results in both early and advanced cases of rheumatoid arthritis. Leflunomide may cause birth defects, so pregnant women are not advised to take this medication.

Synvisc and Hyalgan

In 1998, the FDA granted approval for Synvisc and Hyalgan, known generically as sodium hyaluronate, to be marketed as a pain relief medication for osteoarthritis sufferers. Sodium hyaluronate is a cushioning fluid normally found in the knees, but is lacking in knees afflicted with osteoarthritis. An injection of sodium hyaluronate into the affected site can prevent irritation when the bones of the joint rub together. It is a treatment for patients who do not respond well to other painkillers. The treatment consists of three injections during a two-week period.

Other drugs for treating arthritis's symptoms

Beyond the commonly encountered first- and second-line medications for arthritis, recent research has yielded new approaches to coping with the pain and disability that arthritis sufferers face.

SERMs

A new class of drugs has been introduced into the field of arthritis care. These drugs are called selective estrogen receptor modulators. The Mayo Clinic describes SERMs as "designer estrogens" because they mimic the action of estrogen where it's desired, but not where it is not desired. Raloxifene (Evista) is a new drug in this category that may help increase the bone density and blood lipids in post-menopausal women. However, the safety of this medication needs further study.

Muscle relaxants

Cyclobenzaprine, otherwise known by its brand name, Flexeril, is a muscle relaxant that relieves pain, muscle spasms, stiffness, and discomfort, especially for patients who suffer from fibromyalgia. Cyclobenzaprine does not effect muscle function. This medication is prescribed for short-term use, approximately two to three weeks. Side effects may include:

- Dry mouth.
- Dizziness.

Bright Idea
If you have poor eyesight, ask your pharmacist for oversized, easy-to-open bottles with large print labels. If you have difficulty opening your prescription bottle, ask for a bottle that is not childproof.

- Swelling of the lips, face, or tongue.

- Drowsiness.

Tumor necrosis factor (TNF)

Scientists have recently uncovered an important cause of rheumatoid arthritis that has lead to a new treatment medication. The tumor necrosis factor (TNF) is a protein and chemical messenger that is an important part of the body's normal means to fight infections and injuries. During chronic illnesses, the body may overproduce TNF to harmful levels. In turn, these high levels can exacerbate the symptoms of a chronic illness, such as rheumatoid arthritis. Scientists are currently working on TNF blockers, or inhibitors, that can restrain the TNF before it causes any damage. Enbrel is the first such inhibitor that has been approved by the Food and Drug Administration. Enbrel eliminates, or "soaks up," excess TNF before it can damage joints. Another potential TNF inhibitor, Remicade, is currently under review. Enbrel is approved for use in combination with methotrexate.

Antimalarial drugs

Antimalarial medications stop the growth of malaria, but have also been helpful in treating rheumatoid arthritis. The most commonly prescribed antimalarial medication is hydroxychloroquine, also known by its brand name, Plaquenil.

Side effects may include:

- Upset stomach.

- Skin rashes.

- Muscle weakness.

- Vision changes (rare side effect).

Calcium channel blockers

Raynaud's phenomenon is a reaction of the body to cold exposure. Calcium channel blockers dilate the small blood vessels and relax the muscles to help blood flow to your extremities, such as your hands and feet. Calcium channel blockers are drugs that prevent calcium from entering smooth muscle cells, which causes the smooth muscles to relax and reduces muscle spasms.

Tricyclic antidepressants

Tricyclic antidepressants are prescribed to help those diagnosed with fibromyalgia. To improve your sleep, especially deep sleep, which is vital to fibromyalgia patients, physicians will prescribe tricyclic antidepressants. Tricyclic antidepressants are also called CNS depressants, which means that they slow down the central nervous system and may possibly cause drowsiness. Of course, antidepressants are traditionally used to treat depression, but tricyclic antidepressants can boost serotonin levels. Higher serotonin levels can relieve muscle pain and spasms and help relieve some fibromyalgia symptoms. Commonly prescribed antidepressants include:

- Amitriptyline: more commonly known by its brand name Elavil or Endep. Amitriptyline improves the quality and the depth of sleep, rather than the mood. Amitriptyline is usually taken before bedtime and should be taken with food.

- Fluoxetine: more commonly known by its brand name Prozac. In the last ten years, Prozac has been touted as the cure-all for depression. Prozac works by effecting the chemical

Timesaver
If your arthritis is giving you pain in the joints of your hands, make a point of stocking up on pain relievers that are packaged *without* a child-protector cap. Those can be too hard to open just when you need pain relief the most.

messengers within the brain, called neurotransmitters. It is possible that an imbalance in these neurotransmitters is the cause of depression. Some FMS patients may not be able to tolerate Prozac; ask your doctor about alternatives.

Some minor side effects of the tricyclic antidepressants include:

- Blurred vision.
- Drowsiness.
- Dizziness.
- Weight gain.
- Dry mouth.
- Fuzzy headedness.

Do not stop taking these medications suddenly unless instructed by a physician. Some antidepressants, such as Prozac, need to be slowly weaned from your body.

Protecting your stomach
If you are at high-risk for gastrointestinal complications caused by NSAIDs and aspirin, there may be relief in sight. Arthrotec and Cox-2 inhibitors are two recent advances made to help combat the gastrointestinal distress that the NSAIDs can cause.

Arthrotec
Diclofenac sodium, also known by its brand name Arthrotec, received U.S. marketing clearance from the Food and Drug Administration to treat osteoarthritis patients who are at a high risk for ulcers and other complications caused by NSAIDs. Arthrotec consists of an enteric-coated core containing diclofenac sodium and misoprostol. Arthrotec has side effects that include:

- Birth defects.
- Abdominal pain.
- Diarrhea.
- Stomach upset.

It is, however, believed that these side effects are not as great as those caused by NSAIDs.

Cox-2 inhibitors

Cox-2 inhibitors are another new class of painkillers that promise to cause fewer gastrointestinal side effects than NSAIDs and aspirin. Cox-2 is an enzyme that has been found to cause the gastrointestinal distress in the NSAIDs. A Cox-2 inhibitor stops this distress.

Celebrex is the first Cox-2 inhibitor approved by the FDA for treatment. Studies showed that patients taking Celebrex had a substantially lower risk of ulcers compared to patients who took other NSAIDs.

In 1999, the FDA was also reviewing Vioxx, another Cox-2 inhibitor, with the expectation that additional information on Vioxx would be made available sometime later that year.

Antibiotics

The medical community is still undecided about whether arthritis, specifically rheumatoid arthritis, is triggered by an infection and can be treated with antibiotics. Some believe that if an infection triggered arthritis, antibiotic treatments would have eliminated the bacteria. But it didn't: Rheumatoid arthritis is not curable. The supporters of antibiotic treatment believe that research has shown antibiotics to have some effect in treating rheumatic diseases and that is enough to prove their case.

While the debate goes on, the most talked about antibiotic treatment today is minocycline, a medication from the tetracycline family that was originally used to treat acne. When treating arthritis, minocycline is believed to block metalloproteinases, enzymes that destroy cartilage inside joints. Minocycline is also believed to suppress the immune system. Rheumatologists are uncertain how the antibiotic works, but it appears to reduce the joint swelling and tenderness in some patients. Minocycline is a gentle medication that has a few side effects, including:

- Splotches of dark patches on the skin.
- Dizziness.

The final decision about whether or not you will use antibiotic therapy should be made by your physician and you. Antibiotics will not work for everyone and treatment must be individualized. Once the antibiotic medication is stopped, the benefits will stop too. If your physician prescribes antibiotics for your arthritis pain:

- Ask whether or not the medication should be taken with food or on an empty stomach.
- Women should be aware that antibiotics can cause yeast infections.
- Avoid direct sunlight.
- Be aware that you may experience diarrhea.

Gout treatment

Gout is caused by an excess of uric acid in the blood. Colchicine, allopurinol, and sulfinpyrazone are some of the medications used to prevent gout attacks by decreasing the amount of uric acid in the blood.

Side effects of these medications include:

- Stomach and bowel pain.
- Bloody diarrhea.
- Anemia.
- Nerve disorders.
- Liver failure.
- Hair loss.

Patient education

When your doctor prescribes medication for you to take to alleviate your symptoms, your responsibility is to make sure you follow your doctor's orders and take your medication. However, your responsibility goes beyond just remembering to take your medications. You need to understand what medications you are taking and the importance of taking these medications properly.

Talk to your physician

When your physician prescribes a medication for you, find out as much information as you can about it. Make sure you ask your physician:

- What is the name of the medication? Many medications have similar names. If you are unsure of the name of the medication, have your physician write it down clearly.

- What are the side effects? All medications cause side effects and knowing what you might expect will help you to recognize any potential problems.

- How long do I need to stay on this medication? Do you need to finish the entire prescription, take the medication until you feel better, or call your physician after taking the medication for a certain period of time?

Watch Out!
Do not continue taking anti-rheumatic drugs if you are pregnant or intend to become pregnant. These drugs can cross the placenta and effect the normal development of the fetus. As a result, they may cause birth defects. Also, if you are pregnant, notify your doctor before any x-rays are taken or medications are prescribed.

Moneysaver
Medications can
be expensive,
especially if you
are on a fixed
income and must
pay for your
medication out
of your own
pocket. To help
offset these
costs, ask your
physician for free
samples, or a
less-expensive
generic equiva-
lent. The phar-
macy may also
offer senior dis-
counts. Contact
your local
Association of
Retired Persons
for information
on ordering med-
ication through
mail order. Be
sure to compare
prices.

- Do I take the medication on an empty stomach or with food? How a medication breaks down may be effected by food or lack of food. Ask your physician whether or not your medication needs food to be effective.

- What if I forget to take a dose? It happens to everyone. You are out and do not have your medicine on you, or perhaps you fall asleep early and forget to take your medication. Should you double the dose at the next sched-uled time? Should you take the missed dose right away?

- Is there a problem combining this medication with my other medications? Remind your doc-tor what medications that you are currently tak-ing, how much and how often. If you have more than one doctor, make sure you inform all of them what prescriptions the other have pre-scribed. Keep a list handy with the names and dosages of the medications, and the names and phone numbers of the physicians.

- If you are refilling the medication, make sure the physician informs you if he is changing the brand, the dosage, instructions, or frequency that you are supposed to take the medication. If so, ask why.

Talk to your pharmacist
When you pick up your prescription, remember that pharmacists are human and can make mistakes, too. Before you leave the store:

- Make sure your name, address and physician's name and address are correct on the medica-tion.

- Make sure the name of the medicine on the package is the same that the physician told you.

- Ask your pharmacist how to take the medication and if there are any special instructions.

- Ask your pharmacist what you should do if you forget to take a dose?

- Ask your pharmacist if there is a problem combining this medication with your other medications. Remind your pharmacist what medications that you are currently taking, how much, and how often. If you visit more than one pharmacy, the pharmacist may not have a complete list of medications that you are currently taking. Keep a list handy with the names and dosages of the medications, and the names and phone numbers of the physicians.

- If you are refilling the medication, make sure the refill medication looks the same as it did before. If not, ask the pharmacist why. The new medication could be a generic version, or the pharmacist may have made a mistake.

Typically, when you receive a prescription, you are given a pamphlet explaining what the medication is that you are receiving, any potential side effects, and how to take the medication. If you do not receive a pamphlet such as this, ask your pharmacist if there is any written information on your medication.

Taking your medication
Once you have started to take your medication:

- Do not share your medication with anyone else and do not take anyone else's medication no matter how much they tell you it has helped them.

Bright Idea
Do not store drugs in the bathroom medicine cabinet. Heat and humidity may cause the medicine to lose its effectiveness. Store all medications in a cool, dry area.

- Notify your doctor immediately if you begin to experience any side effects.

- Contact your physician or pharmacist if you begin to take any additional medications.

A deadly combination

It is potentially dangerous to mix two different medications because of the possible side effects. For example, taking aspirin with medications that thin the blood is dangerous since aspirin also thins the blood. It is important to know how mixing two or more medications may affect you. Keep a current list of all medications that you are taking with you and show your pharmacist. Your pharmacist can make certain that there are no side effects from combining your medications.

TABLE 9.1: MEDICATIONS FOR RELIEF OF ARTHRITIS SYMPTOMS

Generic Versions	Brand Name
MUSCLE RELAXANTS	
cyclobenzaprine	Flexeril
NSAIDs	
etodolac	Lodine
acetylsalicylate	Aspirin
indomethacin	Indocin
naproxen	Aleve, Naprosyn
sulindac	Clinoril
ibuprofen	Advil
	Motrin
	Nuprin
tolmetin	Tolectin
diclofenac	Voltaren
	Cataflam
	Voltaren-XR
GOUT MEDICATIONS	
colchicine	Colchicine

COX-2 INHIBITORS	
celecoxib	Celebrex
DMARDs	
methotrexate	Rheumatrex
	Folex
	Mexate
d-penicillamine	Cuprimine
	Depen
leflunomide	Arava
azathioprine	Imuran
cyclophosphamide	Cytoxan
chlorambucil	Leukeran
cyclosporin	Sandimmune
sulfasalazine	Azulfidine
etanercept	Enbrel
ketoprofen	Orudis
ANTI-DEPRESSANTS	
fluoxetine	Prozac
doxepin	Sinequan
	Adapin
GOLD SALTS	
auranofin	Ridaura
aurothioglucose	Solganal
ANTIMALARIAL DRUGS	
hydroxychloroquine	Plaquenil

Just the facts

- Do not just take any medication prescribed to you; learn about it, what it is meant to do, and what the potential side effects are.

- Be smart when taking your medications; follow your doctor's orders and report any side effects right away.

- Keep a list of all medications you are currently taking, the dosages, and the doctor who prescribed them in your wallet, purse, or car. In a medical emergency you may not be able to provide this information.

- Children have the right to know medications they are taking; teach them to be responsible about medications too.

- Keep all medications locked in a safe box or away from children's reach.

GET THE SCOOP ON...
Arthroscopy ▪ Bone and joint replacements ▪
Preparing for surgery ▪ Recovery ▪
New procedures

Surgical Interventions

You probably have experienced arthritis pain that is persistent and severe enough to interfere with your daily activities. You may have tried medication, physical therapy, massage, and a variety of other treatments to help cope with the discomfort, but it just does not get any better.

Unfortunately, it is an unwelcome fact that not all nonsurgical methods of treatment will successfully decrease or eliminate your arthritis pain. When the pain becomes unbearable and the joint is so weakened and damaged that its use is limited, it may be the right time to discuss surgery as an option.

According to the American Academy of Orthopedics, an orthopedist will perform surgery on arthritic joints when other methods of nonsurgical treatment have failed to alleviate pain or when a joint is damaged and not functioning properly.

What type of surgery your doctor recommends will depend on what type of arthritis you have, its severity, and whether or not you are in good physical condition. An orthopedist may choose to remove the diseased or damaged joint lining, realign the joints, fuse the bone ends of a joint together to prevent motion and relieve pain, or replace the entire joint with an artificial joint.

Surgery may sound like a last resort, but for many people it has brought long-awaited relief to their suffering. Before you jump in and agree to a procedure, however, there are many factors to consider. It is important to understand the risks and recovery process as well. This chapter will educate you about the various types of surgical procedures, the risks involved, and the recuperation process.

Is surgery for you?

The Duke University Medical Center has five primary questions to determine if you are a surgical candidate:

1. Is your pain unacceptable?
2. Do you require narcotic pain relievers?
3. Have you tried all other options to achieve pain relief?
4. Are your goals realistic?
5. Are you in good physical condition?

These are not the only deciding factors in determining whether or not you should be operated on, but they provide a useful starting point from which to begin considering your surgical options. Pain cannot be measured, so it is important to communicate with your practitioner.

Arthroscopy: peeking in at the problem

Arthroscopy is a surgical procedure that examines the interior of a joint with a camera-like instrument that is inserted through small incisions made at the joint. The results of the arthroscopy are used in both diagnosis and treatment of joint abnormalities. Such uses include:

- Diagnosing and treating torn cartilage in the knee or shoulder.

- Reconstructing the ligaments in the knee.

- Removing inflamed joint tissues, also known as a synovectomy. The tissue lining can then be biopsied and examined under a microscope to determine the cause of the inflammation.

- Relieving pressure on the carpal tunnel nerve.

- Removing loose bone or cartilage in knee, shoulder, elbow, ankle, or wrist.

Arthroscopy was developed in the 1960s and today is generally an outpatient procedure. Although it is not an "open" or invasive operation, you will still either be given a general, spinal, or local anesthetic. A surgeon inserts an arthroscope, a small tube that contains optical fibers and lenses, through tiny incisions in the skin and into the joint that is being examined. The tube projects pictures of the joint onto a television monitor for the surgeon to see.

These small incisions in the skin mean less trauma to the joint tissues. This results in less pain and perhaps a quicker recovery as compared to open surgery. If any procedures are done in addition to simply examining the joint, this is called arthroscopic surgery.

To be a good candidate for arthroscopy, you must be in good health, be able to tolerate anesthetic, and have good heart and lung function. Any medical conditions that you have should be under control prior to surgery.

When you are out of surgery, a sterile dressing is placed over the small incisions; keep this dry. You may also have a brace or wrap to help stabilize the joint. It is important to rest and elevate the joint while applying ice packs to minimize the pain and swelling. If the procedure was done on your knees, surgeons will encourage you to put pressure on the joint as soon as possible. After surgery, you will begin an exercise program that strengthens the muscles surrounding the joint. It is important to regain stability of the joint as quickly as possible while preventing buildup of scar tissue.

The American Academy of Orthopedic Surgeons reminds patients that "people who have arthroscopy can have different diagnoses and pre-existing conditions, so each patient's arthroscopic surgery is unique to that person. Recovery time will reflect that individuality."

Hemicallotasis: break a leg

Go ahead, break your leg. But don't hit the slopes to do it; just ask your doctor. It sounds strange, but to help eliminate pain caused by arthritic knees, Temple University Hospital surgeons are intentionally fracturing patients' leg bones and then letting the patients pull apart the fracture one millimeter a day. As the fracture widens, new bone grows in the crack and fills it in.

The purpose of this relatively new and still experimental procedure, called hemicallotasis, is to shift a patient's weight from the area in the knee where cartilage has worn away to the knee that still has its cartilage. Arthritic knees usually occur when cartilage wears away between bone. This causes the bones to rub against each other. If the cartilage has worn away on the part of the knee that bears the brunt of a person's weight, the pain is even worse.

Surgeons intentionally create a fracture on the side of the leg in which the cartilage has worn away.

They then insert screws into the bone on either side of the fracture and connect them with a rod. Over a period of three weeks, the patient will turn a dial on the rod once a day. This expands the rod and pulls the fracture open by one millimeter each day. As the fracture grows wider, the patient's bone will naturally grow in the crack and fill it in.

In the past, surgeons would try to achieve the same result by removing a large wedge of bone from the leg. However, this made the person's leg shorter and made it difficult to do a knee replacement if one was needed later. This procedure does not require a cast and allows the patient to begin physical therapy immediately.

Osteotomy

The surgeon may suggest repositioning the joint, a procedure called an osteotomy. This form of treatment is especially recommended for ankylosing spondylitis, when there is a badly bent spine. The surgeon removes damaged bone and tissue and restores the joint to its proper position.

Recovery from an osteotomy is lengthy, perhaps from 6 to 12 months. An osteotomy does not guarantee that the function of the joint will improve. Additional treatment may be necessary. The length of time before another surgery is needed varies greatly and depends on the condition of the joint before the procedure.

Bionic joints

In the 1970s, the escapades of the Bionic Man and Bionic Woman (portrayed by actors Lee Majors and Lindsay Wagner) captured the imaginations of American television audiences. As a result of massive injuries, these two characters received an impressive array of artificial body parts.

For years, these remarkable television heroes combated evil forces: Her bionic legs carried her faster than airplanes his bionic eye saw infrared and was sharper than an eagle's her arm was strong enough to halt a moving train, and he could leap to amazing heights when the situation demanded it. This was science fiction 20 years ago, but better joints through science have become a reality.

Thanks to modern technology, artificial replacements for some parts of the body are now commonplace. The American Academy of Orthopedic Surgeons reports that an estimated 4 million Americans are already carrying artificial joints, and their numbers are increasing as the population ages. The National Center for Health Statistics states that almost 300,000 total hip and knee replacements (the most common artificial joint procedures) are performed annually in the United States. It is quite obvious that the future is here.

The goal of artificial joint replacement is to relieve pain, improve mobility, and improve joint function. A physical examination, laboratory tests, and x-rays will give a clear indication of the extent of your joint damage. Total joint replacement will be considered if other treatment options do not relieve your pain and disability.

Hip replacement

Hip replacement, or arthroplasty, is a surgical procedure that removes the diseased parts of the hip joint and replaces them with new, artificial parts.

The most common reason that people have hip replacement surgery is that the hip joint has worn down from osteoarthritis, rheumatoid arthritis, avascular necrosis (loss of bone caused by insufficient blood supply), injury, or bone tumors.

Unofficially... Bo Jackson won college football's Heisman Trophy and was the first player ever to be chosen both for baseball's All-Star game and football's Pro Bowl. Sadly, at 28 years old, his sports career ended when he was diagnosed with avascular necrosis, a degenerative bone condition, in his left hip. Jackson had a successful artificial hip replacement and is an inspiration, but has never returned to sports.

In the past, hip replacement surgery was an option reserved for people over 60. Typically, this group was less active and put less strain on the artificial hip than younger, more active people. In recent years, however, doctors have found that hip replacement surgery can be very successful in younger patients as well. New technology has improved the artificial components, allowing them to withstand more stress and strain. One study over the last two decades demonstrated the success of total hip replacement surgery in patients under age 30.

That study, conducted by the Centre for Hip Surgery (Lancaster, England), involved 21 males and 34 females with an average age of 24.9 years. Before surgery, most of the patients were severely disabled from hip disease. Younger patients were traditionally thought to be at a higher risk of the loosening and failure of implants, but the study showed that improvements in cementing techniques, implant materials, and prosthetic designs helped the joints to last longer.

A more important factor than age in determining the success of hip replacement is the overall health and activity level of the patient.

An anatomy lesson

The hip joint is basically a ball-and-socket arrangement that allows you to sit, stand, and walk. The hip joint is located where the upper end of the thighbone meets the cup-like structure in the pelvis called the acetabulum. The thighbone looks like a long stem with a ball on the end.

Once the diseased parts of the hip joint have been successfully removed, a prosthesis, or replacement joint, is inserted. The prosthesis can be made

Watch Out!
If you suffer from severe muscle weakness or Parkinson' s disease, you are more likely to damage or dislocate an artificial hip. Patients at a high risk for infections or in poor health are also less likely to recover successfully. As a result, doctors may not recommend hip replacement surgery for these patients.

Note! ➜
The hip and
shoulder are
"ball and socket"
joints. The
rounded top of a
long bone (thigh
or arm) fits into
the socket (at
hip or shoulder)
for maximum
rotation and
mobility.

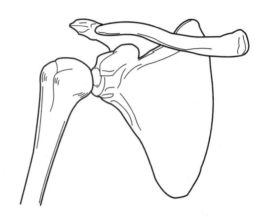

of metal and plastic. In the 1980s, orthopedic surgeons were only able to replace a hip joint with metal parts fixed into place with bone cement. This special glue would bond the new parts of the hip joint to the existing, healthy bone. This is referred to as a "cemented" procedure, developed about 40 years ago. Research has proven the effectiveness of cemented prostheses to reduce pain and increase joint mobility. Cemented replacements are more frequently used than cementless ones for older, less active people and people with weak bones, such as those who have osteoporosis. However, over time the cement begins to crack, causing the artificial parts to loosen.

Cemented or uncemented?

Twenty years ago, scientists addressed the problem with cracking in cemented replacements by developing uncemented prostheses. In an uncemented procedure, the artificial parts are made of porous material. The patient's own bone grows into the pores to form the bond that holds the new parts in place.

An uncemented prosthesis may last longer than cemented replacements because there is no cement that can break away. If a patient needs an additional hip replacement, also known as a revision, the surgery may be easier if the person has an uncemented prosthesis.

The primary disadvantage of an uncemented prosthesis is the extended recovery period. Because it takes a long time for the natural bone to grow and attach to the prosthesis, people with uncemented replacements must limit their activities for up to three months to protect the hip joint. The process of natural bone growth also can cause thigh pain for several months after the surgery.

Studies have also shown that after 10 years, artificial joints without cement had a higher rate of implant mechanical failure as well as a higher revision rate to compensate for loosening. Another approach is using a combination of a cemented thigh bone and a uncemented acetabular—this is known as a "hybrid" prosthesis. At present, cemented prostheses enjoy the greatest success rate.

Because each medical condition is unique, you and your doctor must work together to weigh the advantages and disadvantages and to decide which type of prosthesis is best for you.

Knee replacements

The procedure called "total knee arthroplasty" involves replacing the damaged cartilage of the knee only, and resurfacing the bones of the knee joint with a metal and plastic prosthesis.

The indications for a total knee replacement are almost the same as for a hip replacement: severe pain, significant loss of mobility, and the inability to perform reasonable routine and recreational activities.

Unofficially... According to the American Academy of Orthopedists, almost five million people visit orthopedic surgeons in the United States each year because of knee problems. More than three million of the visits are injury-related; the rest are due to arthritis or other illnesses. In 1994, there were more than 300,000 knee procedures done in the United States.

Note! ➜
The hinge joints
of the knee,
elbow, ankles,
and digits permit
backward and
forward move-
ment of two
articulated bones

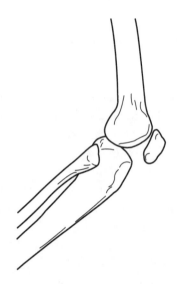

A patient with a knee replacement should expect the joint to last for at least 10 to 20 years. You can maximize the odds for a successful knee replacement by staying at your ideal weight, exercising, protecting against infection, and avoiding impact sports.

Are two better than one?

It might sound sensible to have both knees replaced simultaneously to shorten your hospital stay and recovery time, as well as saving money. Unfortunately, medical studies have shown that serious complications of total knee replacement surgery are more likely to occur when a person has both knees replaced at the same time. Again, discuss this with your surgeon.

Other joints

Although knees and hips are common joint replacements, there are over 2,000 wrist implants and 7,000 hand and finger implants inserted each year as well, according to the *Journal of the American Medical Association.*

There are also artificial shoulder joints. There is no pressure on the shoulder joint, so this is considered a lifetime replacement. The ball in the ball-and-socket joint is replaced, but the socket is rarely replaced. The procedure is either overnight or outpatient, and no cement is used.

Complications

There are risks to every operation, and joint replacement surgery comes with its own set of risks. They include:

- **Dislocation:** According to the American Academy of Orthopedic Surgeons, approximately 120,000 hip replacement operations are performed each year in the United States and less than 10 percent require further surgery. New technology and advances in surgical techniques have greatly reduced the risks involved with hip replacements.

  The most common problem that may happen soon after hip replacement surgery is hip dislocation. The artificial ball and socket are smaller than the normal ones and the ball can become dislodged from the socket if the hip is placed in certain positions. The most dangerous position usually is pulling the knees up to the chest.

- **Inflammation:** Particles can wear off of the artificial joint and be absorbed by the surrounding tissues, causing inflammation. This inflammation may trigger the action of special cells that eat away some of the bone, causing the implant to loosen. If this occurs, doctors may prescribe anti-inflammatory medications or recommend

Moneysaver
If you are a smoker and need a joint replacement, consider quitting first. According to the American Academy of Orthopedic Surgeons, smokers' joint replacement costs average $28,947 compared to $22,019 for nonsmokers. Surgery on smokers also takes longer (153 vs. 112 minutes). Smokers are also more difficult to anesthetize and may require pulmonary consultation.

Bright Idea
In a study done by Indiana University, investigators found that patients who had a better mental health status appeared to improve the most physically after receiving a knee replacement. A positive attitude helps in recovery. If you are scared or depressed about the surgery or the condition, discuss it with your surgeon.

revision surgery. Medical scientists are experimenting with new materials that last longer and cause less inflammation.

- **Phlebitis** (blood clots of a vein): Blood clots may result from several factors, but most frequently from the decreased mobility in your leg that causes a sluggish movement of the blood through the veins. Blood clots may be suspected if pain and swelling develop in your calf or thigh. If this occurs, your orthopedic surgeon may consider tests to evaluate the veins of your leg. Several measures may also be used to reduce the possibility of blood clots, including:

    blood thinning medications (anticoagulants)

    enoxaparin sodium, otherwise known as Lovenox, for blood-clot prevention following hip replacement surgery

    elastic stockings

    exercises to increase blood flow in the leg muscles

    plastic boots that inflate with air to compress the muscles in your legs

Despite the use of these preventive measures, blood clots may still occur. If you develop swelling, redness, or pain in your leg following discharge from the hospital, you should contact your orthopedic surgeon.

- **Damage to blood vessels or nerves:** Nerves around the joint replacement may be damaged during the total replacement surgery. This is more likely to occur when the surgery involves correction of major joint deformity or lengthening of a shortened limb due to an arthritic deformity. Over time these nerve injuries often improve and may completely recover.

- **Unequal leg lengths:** This is a complication that follows total hip replacement. If patients have an obvious difference in their leg lengths, it needs to be corrected.

Revision surgery

Hip replacement is one of the most successful orthopedic surgeries performed—more than 90 percent of people who have hip replacement surgery will never need revision surgery. However, because more young people are having hip replacements, and wearing away of the joint surface becomes a problem after 15 to 20 years, revision surgery is becoming more common. However, revision surgery is more difficult than first-time hip replacement surgery, and the outcome is generally not as good, so it is important to explore all available options before having additional surgery.

Doctors consider revision surgery for two reasons:

1. If medication and lifestyle changes do not relieve pain and disability.

2. If x-rays of the hip show that damage has occurred to the artificial hip that must be corrected before it is too late for a successful revision. This surgery is usually considered only when bone loss, wearing of the joint surfaces, or joint loosening shows up on an x-ray. Other possible reasons for revision surgery include fracture, dislocation of the artificial parts, and infection.

Less common complications of hip replacement surgery include infection, blood clots, and

Unofficially...
Hugh Downs, a co-host on ABC's 20/20, had a double knee replacement in 1997. Over the years, a golf ball had smashed his right kneecap, his left knee had been mangled in a car accident, and he had been thrown from horses, which resulted in water on the knee. Downs had successful double knee surgery and can now ride his horses again and walk without limping.

heterotopic bone formation (bone growth beyond the normal edges of bone).

Preparing for the hospital

Whether you are going in the hospital for the day or for a week, you should be prepared and know what to expect, including:

- When you will be admitted to the hospital? What time do you need to be at the hospital to get settled in?

- What should you bring with you? Do you need special clothes or shoes? Should you bring any medications you are taking? Make sure you leave jewelry and large sums of money at home. Take only enough money to purchase small items from vending machines or the hospital store.

- When will you be going home? Do you need to have someone take you to and from the hospital?

The hospital will probably ask you to sign insurance papers and provide you with a packet of information about your stay in the hospital. If you do not receive a packet, ask the hospital before the day of surgery.

Preparing for surgery

There are many things you can do before and after your operation to make everyday living easier and to help speed your recovery:

- Learn what to expect before, during, and after surgery.

- Arrange for someone to help you around the house for a week or two after coming home from the hospital.

Bright Idea
Inform your orthopedic surgeon about any medical conditions that might affect the surgery. Bring a list of medications and the dosages that you are currently taking to the hospital. This information is important to prevent any potential consequences of combining more than one medication.

- Arrange for transportation to and from the hospital.

- Place items you use every day at arm level to avoid standing up or bending down.

- Prepare food in advance, such as frozen casseroles or soups, which can be reheated and served easily.

- Follow the doctor' s instructions after surgery.

- Work with the physical therapist or other health care professional to rehabilitate your hip.

Recovery and rehabilitation

For joint replacement surgery, you will spend at least 10 days in the hospital, but it may take three to six months to fully recover. This will depend on the type of surgery, your overall health, and the success of rehabilitation.

You will not be able to move too much after surgery. Your hip will be braced with pillows or a special device that will hold your hip in its correct position. There will be a tube to drain fluid and a catheter may be used to drain urine until you can use the bathroom.

In general, the orthopedist will encourage you to use your new joint shortly after your operation. After total hip or knee replacement you will stand and begin to walk with assistance about one to two days after surgery. Do not get discouraged about your progress; take it slow. Initially, you will walk with a walker, crutches, or a cane.

In addition to learning to use your new joint, there are a few other things you can do to facilitate your own recovery. These include:

- **Pain management:** You'll be given medications for pain (and we discuss them in greater detail

Bright Idea
Many hospitals that perform joint replacement surgeries offer preoperative informational classes to help you prepare for surgery. Here you can meet others who are going through joint replacement surgery. You can ask specific questions about your stay in the hospital and your recovery. You will also learn what your limitations are and what your role is in recovery.

in Chapter 9), but there are other, non-medicinal ways to cope with swelling and discomfort after surgery. Swelling is normal in and around the joint after surgery. To decrease swelling, elevate the joint and apply ice packs. You will probably have some temporary pain in the replaced joint. The surrounding muscles are weak from inactivity and the tissues are healing, but the pain should end in a few weeks or months. If you are in severe pain or suspect there may be something wrong, contact your doctor immediately.

■ **Exercise:** Proper exercise can reduce joint pain and stiffness and increase flexibility and muscle strength. Some recommended exercises are cross-country skiing, swimming, walking, and stationary bicycling. These exercises can increase muscle strength and cardiovascular fitness without injuring the new hip. Exercise is an important part of the recovery process. Your orthopedic surgeon or the staff will discuss an exercise program for you after surgery. This varies for different joint replacements and for differing needs of each patient.

After your surgery, you may be permitted to take part in light activities such as golf or walking, but more strenuous sports, such as tennis or running, may be discouraged.

The motion of your joint will generally improve after surgery. The extent of improvement will depend on how stiff your joint was before the surgery.

A physical therapist will teach exercises, such as contracting and relaxing certain muscles that will strengthen the hip. The new hip has a more limited

Watch Out!
Talk to your doctor or physical therapist about developing an appropriate exercise program. Most exercise programs begin with safe range-of-motion activities and muscle strengthening exercises. The doctor or therapist will decide when you can move on to more demanding activities. Many doctors recommend avoiding high-impact activities, such as basketball, jogging, and tennis. These activities can damage the new hip or cause loosening of its parts.

range of movement than a non-diseased hip. Therefore, you will need to be taught how to properly bend and sit to prevent injury to the new hip. As early as one to two days after surgery, you may be allowed to sit on the edge of the bed, stand, and even walk with assistance.

Finding a surgeon and hospital

An orthopedic surgeon is a medical doctor with extensive training in the diagnosis and nonsurgical, as well as surgical, treatment of the musculoskeletal system, including bones, joints, ligaments, tendons, muscles, and nerves.

The American Academy of Orthopedic Surgeons maintains a list of physicians who are specialists in problems of the hip and provides physician referrals by geographic area. (Check Appendix B, "Resources," for how to contact them.)

When you meet your orthopedic surgeon, get to know his or her background. Ask:

- Where did you go to medical school?
- What year did you graduate?
- Where was your residence and what year was it completed?
- Are you board certified?
- How many years have you been in practice?

It is also important to ask if the surgeon receives any benefits, money or otherwise, from any orthopedic manufacturer.

You should also ask questions about the surgical procedure, such as:

- Will you be performing the joint procedure alone or with the assistance of a resident or fellow?

- Will you be in the operating room with me for the entire procedure?

- Will you be the one making all of the bone cuts and aligning the implants?

- Are the implants you are using part of a study? Have the implants you intend to use been in use in the U.S. for at least five years?

Feeling comfortable at the hospital is just as important as feeling comfortable with the doctor, so check both out thoroughly. Ask for written information about the hospital's experience with joint replacement surgery. Also, make sure the hospital is accredited by The Joint Commission on Accreditation of Healthcare Organizations (JCAHO). The JCAHO is the nationwide authority that surveys hospitals and decides whether a hospital gets, keeps, or loses accreditation based on its meeting certain criteria for staffing, equipment, and facility safety requirements. Although accreditation is voluntary, most hospitals go through the process. If the hospital that you are considering is not accredited, it is important to know why.

Long term outlook

In 90 percent of total joint replacement procedures, the new joint will last 10 years; 80 percent can be expected to last 20 years. However, research still needs to be conducted and implants need more improvement. Nonetheless, patients are already enjoying what modern technology has done for them.

This does not mean that the scientific community will stop here. There are other less drastic procedures currently being studied that may one day take the place of joint replacement surgery.

Cartilage cell transplantation

Artificial joint replacement surgery has been very successful, but replacing your joints is really not the ultimate goal of the medical community. Scientists would prefer that the human body make what it needs to keep the original joint healthy. Scientists are currently researching ways for the body to regenerate its own tissue and cartilage in the bone.

The process, called cartilage cell transplantation, means removing healthy cells from one area of the body, multiplying them, and growing new cartilage in a laboratory. Then the healthy new cartilage is transplanted back into your body, replacing the diseased cells with these healthy ones.

The surgery is currently performed only on patients who have been diagnosed in the early stages of arthritis. It is also only being done on ankles and knees, not hips since the hip requires a major operation to expose the joint. Scientists hope that one day cartilage cell transplantation might prevent the need for joint replacement surgery.

Joint restoration

Joint restoration is another minimally invasive technique that may one day provide relief for millions of osteoarthritis sufferers. Joint restoration means applying a liquid joint polymer to the joint surface. This polymer restores the bone surface and allows the bones to glide smoothly against each other. More tests are needed on this procedure.

Experts have estimated that in a few decades 1 in 12 people will have an artificial body part. Although we are not up to par with the Bionic Woman yet, those with crippling diseases who have been freed from pain are heralding joint replacement surgery as one of the century' s greatest medical achievements.

Just the facts

- Exhaust other nonsurgical forms of treatment first.
- Discuss the risks of surgery with your doctor.
- Prepare at home for the recovery process.
- Thinking positive helps the recovery along.

GET THE SCOOP ON...
Acupuncture, acupressure, and arthritis ▪
Herbs ▪ Chiropractors ▪ Finding an alternative
practitioner ▪ Spotting a fraud

Alternative Therapies

A ccording to a study published in the Journal of the American Medical Association, four out of ten Americans used alternative medicine therapies in 1997. Americans also paid an estimated $21.2 billion for services provided by alternative medicine practitioners. The total number of visits to alternative medicine practitioners increased by almost 50 percent since 1990 and exceeded the total number of visits to all U.S. primary care physicians.

Why is there such an increase in the number of Americans turning to alternative therapies, such as herbs, magnets, chiropractors, and acupuncture to treat their illnesses or keep them well? When asked, many patients stated that they use alternative treatments because conventional therapies have not eased or eliminated their symptoms. Other patients said that they want to stop taking synthetic "drugs."

In addition to trying alternative treatments for these reasons, patients who suffer from arthritis may also use alternative treatments to help ease other symptoms, such as headaches that have been caused by the stress of having a chronic illness, or dry skin

213

caused by medications. Combining alternative treatments with prescription treatments ordered by your physician is called complementary alternative medicine, or CAM.

This chapter will examine many different types of alternative treatments from acupressure to magnets, and see if any of these treatments have been proven to relieve arthritis symptoms. Most importantly, this chapter will teach you how to educate yourself about treatments before using them. (See Chapter 8 for more information on experimental medications and therapies.)

The pros and cons of the growing popularity of alternative medicine

Many alternative therapies have actually been in use for thousands of years, such as herbal remedies and acupuncture. However, much of the medical community has been hesitant to approve these treatments for arthritis except in those cases where scientific studies demonstrate their likely effectiveness and safety, especially for long-term users.

Another concern physicians have is that less than 40 percent of the patients surveyed informed their physician that they were using alternative treatments. Physicians are especially concerned because an estimated 15 million Americans in 1997 took prescription medications and herbal remedies at the same time. When alternative therapies are combined with conventional medication, there is an increased risk of side effects and potentially deadly complications. If your physician is not informed when you use alternative therapies, potential problems may not be uncovered.

If you have been diagnosed with, or suffer from, arthritis, alternative treatments may provide some

Unofficially...
In *Nature's Cures*, author Michael Castleman writes, "according to legend...a Chinese soldier had an illness his physicians could not cure. During the fighting, he was hit by an arrow and received a superficial wound. The wound healed and, oddly, so did his illness...ancient Chinese physicians began recording the places where a stab wound caused healing. Their observations became the foundation of acupuncture, acupressure, Shiatsu, and reflexology."

relief of your symptoms. Remember though, no alternative medication or treatment claims to cure arthritis. Instead, these therapies claim to reduce your symptoms. Become educated about any alternative treatments before using them or combining them with your current medications.

Acupressure and acupuncture

Chinese and Japanese practitioners believe in the balance of the internal energy of the body, called the "qi" (pronounced "chi"). It is believed that when your qi levels are low, that is when your body is ill. Acupressure and acupuncture are two methods of raising your qi level back to normal to balance your internal energy and return you to good health.

Acupressure has been used as a Chinese form of hands-on healing for more than 5000 years. Acupressure is the pressing of certain points on the body which would alleviate certain ailments or pain.

Acupuncture has also been around for thousands of years. Acupuncture is the practice of inserting very fine needles into the skin to stimulate certain points in the body. Heat (moxibustion), pressure, friction, suction (cupping), or electromagnetic energy (electro-acupuncture) are used on the needles to stimulate the points as well. Acupuncture and acupressure are similar in that they both use the same points on the body. The difference is that acupuncture uses needles, and acupressure uses gentle yet firm pressure with the hands.

In 1997, the National Institutes of Health (NIH) approved the use of acupuncture for some medical conditions, including the control of pain, nausea, and vomiting caused by chemotherapy,

Timesaver
Want to find an acupuncturist? Contact the American Academy of Medical Acupuncture (AAMA). The organization restricts membership to medical doctors and doctors of osteopathy. Write to 5820 Wilshire Blvd., Suite 500, Los Angeles, CA 90036 or call (213) 937-5514.

postoperative surgery, dental pain, and possibly pregnancy.

The NIH also stated that acupuncture, either alone or in conjunction with other treatments, may help headaches, general muscle pain, low back pain, and carpal tunnel syndrome. A study reported in 1997 by the University of Maryland says that acupuncture may actually play a useful role in the treatment of osteoarthritis of the knee. This treatment, in combination with conventional medical therapy, significantly improved pain and disability. However, neither the NIH nor any other leading medical organizations have released a definitive statement on acupuncture as a treatment for any form of arthritis.

Antioxidants

Antioxidants are compounds that clear oxygen-reactive chemicals, or "free radicals," from the circulation and tissue. These free radicals can lead to disease and tissue damage of your joints. Vitamins C, E, and beta-carotene (or Vitamin A) are also known as antioxidants, as well as several herbs. Eating foods rich in antioxidants can help to reduce this damage to your joints. In 1997, a study from Johns Hopkins University associated foods rich in beta-carotene with a reduced risk of rheumatoid arthritis. The study showed that the beta-carotene levels of the people who had not fallen victim to arthritis were 20 percent higher than those who did.

Aromatherapy

Think about how you feel when you smell mom's apple pie, freshly cut flowers, or the ocean air. It is a known fact that good aromas make us feel good, and that is the philosophy behind aromatherapy. Aromatherapy relies on chemical scents from herbs and extracts and, used with oils, lotions, and candles, is used to relieve pain and stress, and claims to boost the immune system. When you inhale these scents, such as peppermint or lilac, it is believed that the scents stimulate the nervous system and the brain.

Aromatherapy is a fast-growing field of alternative medicine, but it has actually been around for thousands of years, dating back to the ancient Greeks, Romans, and Egyptians. Each oil serves a different purpose. For example, some oils are for relaxation, some for soothing, and some are meant to relieve pain. Aromatherapy has not been scientifically recognized as a treatment for arthritis, but it is a beneficial and harmless way to reduce stress and tension and relax the muscles in your body. This may help to alleviate stiff painful joints.

Chiropractice

Perhaps best known as the doctor who "cracks your back or your neck," chiropractors believe that the state of your health depends on the condition of your musculoskeletal system and your nervous system.

A chiropractor corrects the abnormal positions of your body by manipulating or "adjusting" it into its normal position. A doctor of chiropractic completes premedical studies and four years of training in a school of chiropractics.

Over the last several years, the possible benefits of chiropractic care have been given more recognition. In 1997, the NIH Office of Alternative Medicine and the National Institute of Arthritis and Musculoskeletal and Skin Diseases (NIAMSD) awarded a research grant to support the first study of chiropractic care. Presently, however, there are

66
Have your regular physician recommend a chiropractor. Many physicians now recognize the value of chiropractors. My physician's recommendation gave me more confidence in my chiropractor. I wasn't concerned that the chiropractor was going to hurt me or was treating me for problems I didn't have because I trust my regular doctor's recommendation.
—Susannah, 30
99

Bright Idea
Make sure there is a lifeguard on duty whenever you are in a pool or performing your water exercises. Never exercise alone. Fatigue and muscle cramps can make it difficult to get out of the water quickly and without help. This can put your life in jeopardy.

no studies that address the safety and long-term benefits of chiropractic care for arthritis.

Exercise

Unfortunately, for some arthritis patients, even a simple walk is difficult and possibly painful, so other forms of exercise, such as cycling or stair-climbing are simply out of the question. One form of alternative therapy, however, can benefit all arthritis sufferers.

Water exercises, also called hydrotherapy, is not an easy workout, but when you are in water, your body is buoyant. There is no impact or pressure on your bones or joints. The water reduces the amount of stiffness in the joint. When you move in water, it is painless, but your body actually works harder to get through the water. As a result, you receive painless strength-training benefits. Check out your local YMCA or community swimming pool for more information.

Herbs

An herb is a plant or part of a plant that has medicinal, aromatic, or savory qualities. Although herbs might seem "natural" or lacking in chemicals, all plants actually produce and contain a variety of chemical substances that act upon the body.

Herbs had been used to treat illnesses and injuries to the body for thousands of years. Interest in herbal remedies in the United States is on the rise. According to a report in the Archives of Family Medicine, more than one third of Americans use herbs for health purposes, spending over $3.5 billion annually. Some of the recent popular herbal remedies include St. John's Wort (for depression), ginseng (for energy), and ginkgo biloba (for mental sharpness).

Unfortunately, many Americans who use herbs are not well informed of the efficiency and safety of these products.

Herbal products can only be marketed in the United States as a food supplement. Manufacturers cannot make any health claims on the labeling, or in the advertising of the product, without approval from the Food and Drug Administration.

How do I take herbs?

There are many ways you can take herbs:

■ Extracting the juice from the herbs.

■ Mashing it into a paste (external use).

■ Boiling it down (steeping).

■ Drinking it as a hot or cold tea.

■ Grinding it into a powder and taking it in pill form.

■ Combining it with alcohol or vinegar.

■ Soaking it in an oil.

If you do not know anything about herbs, it is important to ask an herbal specialist, or an herbalist, to help you use these herbs safely. Again, make sure you tell your physician that you are using these treatments so he can research any potential complications.

An herbal round-up

Here we will discuss a few of the most frequently mentioned herbs that manufacturers claim to help treat arthritis symptoms. There are not many studies done on whether herbs help arthritis symptoms, but again this does not mean that you cannot benefit from them.

■ Alfalfa is a seed sprout that has traditionally been used as a source of good nutrition. Alfalfa

Unofficially...
A study done by Warner Lambert showed that nine out of 10 physicians and 96 percent of all pharmacists report a dramatic increase in the interest of their patients in herbal supplements compared to five years ago. 76 percent of health care professionals believe that the use of herbal supplements will continue to grow and they would most likely recommend herbal supplements five years from now.

Unofficially...
In 1964, Norman Cousins, editor of *Saturday Review,* was diagnosed with ankylosing spondylitis, stiffness and inflexibility of the spine. Convinced that positive emotions would speed his recovery, he watched "Candid Camera" and movies by the Marx Brothers and the Three Stooges. He also told jokes and read funny books. His symptoms improved and he went on to document his recovery in *Anatomy of an Illness.*

leaves contain beta-carotene, vitamin K, and several trace minerals, but their link to treating arthritis symptoms has not yet been proven.

- Aloe can be squeezed into fresh juice and applied on sore joints.

- Capsicum/cayenne peppers, contains capsaicin, an irritant that produces a feeling of warmth throughout the body. Once you use capsicum you will begin to sweat. Capsaicin is now available as a salve that has been approved by the FDA for pain relief. It does not cure arthritis, but can help to relieve pain. Cayenne pepper has the same medical reactions that capsicum peppers has but cayenne pepper has not been studied.

- Celery seed is used to treat gout. It is a diuretic and will help to eliminate excess uric acid from the body. It is often mixed with juniper berry.

- Chamomile is commonly used as a sedative, anti-spasmodic, and anti-inflammatory. Chamomile is considered safe by the Food and Drug Administration, with no known side effects when used during pregnancy, during lactation, or in childhood. It is commonly used as a tea or applied as a compress.

- Devil's claw, used as an anti-inflammatory and pain reliever. However, research has not supported the use of devil's claw in alleviating arthritis symptoms. Devil's claw does increase stomach acid, so anyone with gastrointestinal irritations or ulcers, or currently using nonsteroidal anti-inflammatory drugs, should not use the herb.

- Echinacea, also known as purple coneflower and black-eyed Susan, is an immune system booster and an antibiotic, and increases the chances of fighting off illnesses. It stimulates production of T-cells and enhances white blood cell function. However, use of echinacea is discouraged during pregnancy and for people with tuberculosis or autoimmune problems. It stimulates production of T-cells and enhances white blood cell function.

- Feverfew, also known as "featherfew," is used to prevent migraines, and is also being studied as a possible treatment to reduce the symptoms of rheumatoid arthritis. So far, studies reported in the Journal of the American Medical Association show that feverfew did not reduce rheumatoid arthritis symptoms, but additional studies are still being conducted. Side effects from the use of this herb include oral ulcers, headaches, allergic reaction, and gastrointestinal irritation.

- Flaxseed can be cold pressed into its liquid form, which is an oil. It is probably better known for its beneficial effect on cholesterol, but it is also quite effective for relief of arthritic pain.

- Garlic, great for making foods taste great, has antioxidant properties as well. Antioxidants clear oxygen-reactive chemicals, or "free radicals" from the circulation and tissue. These free radicals can be called the "bad guys" that lead to disease and tissue damage. There are no serious side effects of garlic.

- Ginger, another warming herb that has been useful for treating nausea, cramps, and spasms, including menstrual cramps, may help muscle spasms caused by certain forms of arthritis. One

Moneysaver
Not all alternative treatments are covered by your health insurance. Contact your carrier before trying any alternative treatments and obtain, in writing, what treatments are covered and if you are required to pay any deductibles, etc. Save all of your receipts from payments should a question about your treatment arise later.

Watch Out!
If you have severe ragweed allergies you may be allergic to chamomile and other members of this family, including echinacea, feverfew, and milk thistle. Do not use it with other sedatives or alcohol.

study of patients taking an average of 5 grams of fresh ginger or 1 gram of powdered ginger showed reduced signs of inflammation.

- Ginkgo biloba helps the circulation, but the most popular use for this herb is in the effect it has on the brain. It helps memory and brain function.

- Ginseng stimulates the immune system, supports lungs, and lowers blood pressure.

- Juniper berry is a diuretic herb used to treat gout. It may help the body eliminate uric acid. However, prolonged use may actually damage your kidneys, so go easy.

- Meadowsweet is used as an anti-rheumatic and anti-inflammatory. It may also be used to treat gout.

- St. John's Wort is most commonly used as an antidepressant, to treat anxiety and nervous tension. Patients who suffer from chronic pain may suffer from depression, too.

- White willow bark is an ancient remedy used for treating rheumatism and aches and pains. It has been used as a painkiller, anti-inflammatory, and fever-reducer. White willow is the natural form and origin of the modern aspirin, but today's form of aspirin does not contain any form of willow.

- Oil of wintergreen, or methyl salicylate, is used as an active ingredient in many over-the-counter liniments, lotions, or ointments. Applied externally, methyl salicylate can help to reduce the pain and inflammation of acute rheumatism.

According to the Mayo Clinic, the following herbs are definitely toxic and should be avoided:

- Chaparral grows in southwestern United States and Mexico, and has been used in herbal teas without toxicity. In tablet form, however, chaparral has proven to cause toxic hepatitis, including the case of a patient who required a liver transplant.

- Comfrey can cause liver damage and possibly death.

- Ephedra (ma huang) is being used as a weight loss aid, although there is no reliable evidence that the active agent, ephedrine, is safe or effective in aiding weight loss. Ephedrine increases blood pressure. It can cause heart palpitations and can lead to stroke. It has been linked to the deaths of at least 15 people.

- Lobelia, also called Indian tobacco, can cause vomiting, convulsions, coma, and death.

- Yohimbe, promoted as an aphrodisiac, can cause weakness, paralysis, gastrointestinal problems, and even psychosis. Yohimbine is sometimes prescribed in the United States for treatment of impotence. However, self-medication is strongly discouraged because of its side effects.

Homeopathy

When an infant receives an immunization for polio, that baby is receiving a smaller form of the disease itself. The body develops antibodies or an immunity to the disease. Homeopathy is a form of medicine that treats the body to heal itself. The objective is to prevent the patient from getting the illness again.

Watch Out!
The American Medical Association advises patients who are contemplating pregnancy, or are already pregnant or lactating, not to use herbal treatments. Some herbal products may cause premature uterine contractions, and long-term scientific studies have not documented the effect of herbs on an unborn baby or nursing infant.

The theory was advanced in the late 18th century by Dr. Samuel Hahnemann, who believed that a large amount of a particular drug may cause symptoms of a disease and a mild dose may reduce those symptoms; thus, some disease symptoms could be treated by very small doses of medicine. Homeopathy uses animal, vegetable, and mineral preparations to cure a person's illness. Homeopathy individualizes a treatment plan.

Magnets

Moneysaver
Before ordering any magnetic or other alternative products, ask the manufacturer what their return policy is. Can you get your money back, or just credit? Be wary if the company only has a post office box, will not give out information on the product or the company, or does not have a return policy. In most cases, it is a sham.

The Museum of Questionable Medical Devices reports that magnetic bandages were sold in the 1970s as a promise of temporary relief of minor aches and pains of muscles and joints. The claim behind magnets is that when you put the magnet on an affected (or painful) area, electrically-charged elements in the bloodstream are attracted to the magnets. This attraction stimulates blood flow, which would speed the repair to the affected area.

Supporters claim that magnets are supposed to be worn all the time to obtain the maximum benefits. However, magnets should not be used by people who wear a pacemaker, or have surgically implanted metal pins or screws. There are a variety of magnets that you can use: either larger magnets that are wrapped in pads and taped to the skin or smaller pellet-like magnets. Although the medical community has initiated studies on magnetic therapy, there is no conclusive medical evidence at this time there is any benefit to magnetic therapy or a connection to benefiting arthritis patients, though anecdotal evidence is strong.

Nutritional supplements

No one food contains all of the vitamins or minerals that your body needs to stay healthy. Vitamins cannot be made in the body. As a result, you may need to take vitamin supplements. These dietary supplements are sold over-the-counter, but that does not guarantee their safety. Some dietary supplements may have harmful side effects, especially if you combine them with certain foods or prescription medications. It is important to discuss dietary supplements with a registered dietitian and your pharmacist.

- Capsicum peppers: As mentioned previously, capsicum contains an irritant that produces a feeling of warmth throughout the body, which causes you to sweat. It's use is limited to pain relief—it is not a cure. The same is true for cayenne pepper.

- Glucosamine sulfate: Glucosamine is a substance that is synthesized by the body and can play a role in repairing cartilage. It is believed that it may stimulate cartilage cells to grow and may inhibit the enzymes that break down this process.

- Chondroitin: Another natural substance found in cartilage. Supporters claim that combining it with glucosamine boosts the actions of both agents. However, according to the American Academy of Orthopaedic Surgeons, little scientific evidence exists to show that Chondroitin and glucosamine sulfate relieve chronic joint pain. The American College of Rheumatology and the Arthritis Foundation do not recommend glucosamine chondroitin as a treatment for arthritis. Both organizations have publicly stated that further studies are needed before any formal support of the supplement can be made.

▪ Fish oil supplements: Studies have shown that omega-3 fatty acids, a polyunsaturated fat found in fish, may have an anti-inflammatory effect on the body. Researchers believe that omega-3 fatty acids decrease the production of the tumor necrosis factor (TNF), a protein produced in high levels of chronic illness, such as rheumatoid arthritis.

Omega-3 fatty acids can be found in seafood, especially higher-fat fish such as albacore tuna, mackerel, and salmon, or it can be taken as a dietary supplement. Some studies have shown that RA patients who took omega-3 fatty acid supplements experienced significant reduction in pain and swelling, and an improvement in morning stiffness and fatigue. Research is still being conducted to see if omega-3 fatty acids can be an alternative to NSAIDs. However, the American Dietetic Association states that fish oil supplements that contain omega-3 fatty acids are not recommended as a substitute for fish, or as a dietary supplement. The side effects of omega-3 fatty acids are minimal, consisting largely of nausea, flatulence, and diarrhea.

Patient education

In a 1995 article published in *Arthritis & Rheumatism*, researchers had analyzed dietary supplements called "Chinese black balls" (known by brand names Miracle Herb and Tung Shueh) after five people developed stomach pain or drowsiness. The only ingredients listed on the product are herbs, but the analysis revealed the presence of NSAID medications and benzodiazepines, anti-anxiety medications such as Valium and Librium.

Since the patients did not know that these medications were in this product, one patient was taking twice the recommended NSAID dosage by combining her herbal pills with her prescription NSAIDs. This left her at a dangerously high risk for gastrointestinal bleeding and ulcers.

Chuifong toukuwan is another Chinese herbal medication that was promoted as an arthritis cure. Unfortunately, in 1980, according to the Food and Drug Administration, several illnesses and deaths were linked to use of this product.

Do you know what you are taking? Many herbal medications have side effects, and potential drug interactions when combined with prescription and over-the-counter medications that you may not know about. For example, combining corticosteroids with echinacea may offset the immunosuppressive effects of the corticosteroids. If you are using nonsteroidal anti-inflammatory drugs as well as herbs, you may also suffer from additional gastrointestinal irritation. As a result, it is vital to apprise your physician of all the treatments you are using to help reduce your arthritis symptoms. Keep a list, and be sure to note dosages, frequency, and any side effects.

Make sure you are educated about any product that you use, but do not feel foolish about falling for a gimmick. Many smart, educated consumers are lured into buying or trying products by suggestive wording, promises of cures, and inexpensive investments. The Food and Drug Administration estimates that 38 million Americans have used a fraudulent health product within the past year. The most important thing to remember is that there are no miracle cures, so if a practitioner or a

66

I spoke with my doctor, an osteopath, about trying alternative methods. She is very supportive of complementary medicine. Her thoughts were that if it works for you, why not try it? I have found a great relief by using glucosamine/chondroitin.

—Mary Pat, 44

99

manufacturer claims a product is a miracle cure, this is a red flag for fraud. Here are some good questions to keep in your mind before trying any treatments:

- How old is the treatment?
- Have there been any studies done on the treatment, or is it approved by the Food and Drug Administration?
- What are the ingredients?
- What are the side effects?

Before buying a product, keep an eye out for these catch phrases:

- This product cures it all.
- This product promises a quick and easy cure.
- This product is harmless and all-natural.
- The medical community does not accept this product.

That last one is a lulu: Anyone discovering a cure for a serious condition will be taken seriously by the medical community. Claims to the contrary are just efforts to hook you into buying their fraudulent product.

Who is treating you?

Looking for a qualified alternative practitioner was just as important as finding a qualified rheumatologist or primary care physician. Just so you know, here are the different types of alternative practitioners:

- Ayurvedic practitioners believe in using traditional Indian therapies and take a complete-wellness approach to life.
- Chinese medicine practitioners use herbs and bodywork techniques such as acupressure and acupuncture. Chinese practitioners believe in

the qi, or the energy in the body, and increasing this energy increases your illness or symptoms.

■ Environmental practitioners focus on how the environment affects us.

■ Osteopaths are physicians who incorporate chiropractice, traditional techniques, and holistic health in treating bone diseases.

■ Homeopaths are physicians who practice homeopathy.

When you are searching for an alternative practitioner, check the practitioner's background. Here are some tips in finding an alternative practitioner:

1. Ask your physician, friends, or co-workers for a recommendation.

2. Call a medical university for a recommendation. Many have doctor referral offices.

3. Call trade associations and ask for a recommendation.

4. Remember, homeopaths, acupuncturists, acupressurists, and those who practice other forms of homeopathic medicine do NOT need to be licensed. Therefore, it is very difficult to confirm that the person treating you is a qualified professional. Many alternative doctors may also be medical doctors, a doctor of osteopathy (D.O.) a doctor of chiropractic (D.C.) or have other degrees from medical schools that he or she has attended. Ask to see them and make calls to confirm.

5. Plan a consultation and ask questions to determine whether this practitioner will meet your needs.

Bright Idea
To find an osteopath, acupuncturist, or another alternative practitioner, contact the International Association of Healthcare Practitioner Directory, but be sure to follow the advice listed here for finding a practitioner. Call (800) 311-9204 ext. 9359.

6. Ask about tests and methods of treatment. Make sure the practitioner informs you of the side effects of any treatment.

7. Make sure you are comfortable with the practitioner.

8. Ask about their background, such as:

- Are you licensed?
- Do you have a specialty?
- How long have you been in practice?
- Do you have any clients that I can speak to?
- Do you take or file insurance?

Looking ahead

The Office of Alternative Medicine (OAM) was originally established in 1991. Congress mandated that the OAM study seven areas of alternative medicine, including:

- Alternative systems of medical practice.
- Bioelectromagnetic applications.
- Diet.
- Nutrition.
- Lifestyle changes.
- Herbal medicine.
- Manual healing.
- Mind/body control.
- Pharmacological and biological treatments.

Early in 1999, the Office of Alternative Medicine was further developed and changed to the National Center for Complementary and Alternative Medicine (NCCAM). At that time, Congress appropriated $50 million from the 1999 budget to study complementary and alternative therapies.

The medical community is more open-minded to alternative treatments today than they were in the past, but it is still vital to the medical community that alternative treatments are scientifically evaluated.

Just the facts

- Alternative treatments are not cures for arthritis.

- Complementary alternative medicine (CAM) may provide the best treatment for your symptoms.

- It is important to inform your physician of all the treatments you are using for your arthritis.

- Check the background of anyone you use to treat your symptoms.

- If you feel that you are being harmed in any way by an alternative treatment, or are experiencing side effects, stop using the treatment immediately and notify your physician.

Lifestyle Changes to Ease Arthritis

PART IV

GET THE SCOOP ON...
Antioxidants ▪ Consuming calcium for
your bones ▪ Phytochemicals

Chapter 12

Arthritis and Nutrition

Wouldn't it be nice to eat your favorite foods and have them eliminate your arthritis symptoms or, better yet, cure your arthritis? Everyone wishes that all of their medical ailments could be cured by eating a magic food, or popping a magic pill. The sad fact is, however, that arthritis cannot be cured with one food, or one pill.

This chapter will inform you about foods that have been touted as miracle cures, the benefits of eating healthy, and how to start eating right to gain maximum health benefits.

Eating for health

Good nutrition *does* play a part in your health. Without the right vitamins, minerals, carbohydrates, fats, proteins, and water, your body will fail to function properly, and leave you susceptible to illnesses and injuries.

The only form of arthritis that is directly caused by diet is gout. Gout is caused by a high uric acid level in the blood. This is directly related to specific foods, such as seafood, mushrooms, and organ meats. By eliminating these items from your diet, symptoms of gout are often alleviated as well, although medication might still be necessary to keep the symptoms at bay.

While eating or eliminating any one food, might not help your arthritis symptoms, healthy eating as a whole can keep your body fine-tuned. This, in turn, may alleviate some of your symptoms. Healthy eating also helps you lose excess weight, which will relieve extra pressure on your joints and reduce your risk of osteoarthritis.

There have been some advances in the field of nutrition and its link to arthritis. Researchers have uncovered a direct relationship with consuming antioxidants and omega-3 fish oils and reducing symptoms of arthritis. This is just a start, however, and other foods are still being researched. In the meantime, eating a healthy, balanced diet and maintaining a healthy weight is always a win-win situation.

Antioxidants

In the late 1980s, researchers in Framingham, Massachusetts conducted a study on more than 100 patients who had osteoarthritis. The researchers suggested that a diet rich in certain vitamins and nutrients, particularly vitamins C, D, and E, may actually slow the progression of osteoarthritis, then documented what these patients ate for an entire year.

The study concluded that the patients who ate more foods that were rich with these vitamins had significantly lowered their chances of having their disease progress. The patients who had a high level of vitamin C had reduced the progression of the disease by two-thirds. Those with a high level of vitamin D had reduced the progression of the disease by three-fourths, and those who had a high level of vitamin E reduced their progression by one-half.

Are these miracle vitamins? No, not really, but go ahead and call them the "good guys" in your body. Vitamins C, E, and beta-carotene (or vitamin A) are known as antioxidants. These compounds have a special job of clearing oxygen-reactive chemicals, or "free radicals," from the circulation and tissue. These free radicals can be called the "bad guys" that lead to disease and tissue damage. Eating foods rich in antioxidants can help to reduce this damage to your joints. While vitamin D is not an antioxidant, it plays a key role in promoting bone growth and strength and is vital in keeping our joints healthy.

Almost a decade later, in 1997, a study from Johns Hopkins University associated foods rich in beta-carotene with a reduced risk of rheumatoid arthritis. Researchers analyzed frozen blood samples of 20,000 people that were taken a few years before. The study showed that the beta-carotene levels of the people who had not fallen victim to arthritis were 20 percent higher than those who did.

Antioxidants are beneficial, but as I will say repeatedly in this chapter, they are not the only nutrients that we need for strong bones and a healthy body. Right now, let's take a look at each of these antioxidants individually and see exactly what part they play in your body, and what foods you need to eat to benefit from these vitamins.

Vitamin A

Vitamin A promotes the growth of cells and tissues in your body. A significant deficiency of vitamin A, in turn, may lead to poor growth. Vitamin A also

Bright Idea
The easiest way
to remember
what foods are
rich in antioxi-
dants is to
remember colors.
Red, yellow,
orange and many
dark green leafy
vegetables, are
loaded with cru-
cial antioxidants.

helps you see clearer ("eat your carrots") and is a precursor to beta-carotene. Too much vitamin A, however, can actually lead to reduced bone density and increase your risk of osteoporosis. Some sources of vitamin A include:

Dark green leafy vegetables

Liver

Sweet potatoes

Eggs

Milk fortified with vitamin A

Oranges

Vitamin C

Vitamin C helps to produce collagen, a connective tissue that holds muscles, bones, and other tissues together. Vitamin C also helps form and repair red blood cells, bones, and tissues. Furthermore, vitamin C is known as the vitamin to beat colds, but while nothing can prevent a cold, vitamin C does helps to protect you from infection by keeping your immune system healthy.

A deficiency of vitamin C can cause scurvy, a disease that causes mouth ulcers and bleeding. Many people can, however, take too much of a good thing. Too much vitamin C, taken at doses of 500 milligrams or more per day, can cause genetic damage and lead to cancer or trigger rheumatoid arthritis, according to a study by the University of Leicester, in the U.K. Think citrus when you are looking for some sources of vitamin C:

Oranges

Grapefruits

Kiwi

Black currants

Papaya

Red peppers

Broccoli

Brussel sprouts

Vitamin D

Vitamin D helps the body absorb two other important minerals—calcium and phosphorus (more on them later). Unfortunately, as we age, our body's ability to produce vitamin D gradually diminishes, but eating foods rich in vitamin D can make up the difference. Not enough vitamin D puts you at risk for osteoporosis. Children who lack vitamin D can develop rickets, or defective bone growth.

Too much vitamin D may lead to kidney stones or damage, weak muscles and bones, and excessive bleeding. Sources of vitamin D include:

Egg yolks

Liver

Fish

A walk in the sun for 10 or 15 minutes a few times a week will also provide you with the necessary requirements

Vitamin E

Vitamin E has been in the news recently because of its benefit of reducing the risk of heart disease and cancer. It is rare to be vitamin E deficient. According to the American Dietetic Association, the two exceptions are premature, very low birth weight infants, and individuals that do not absorb fat normally. Too much vitamin E does not cause any major symptoms, but the ADA states that it does not cause any major benefits either. Sources of vitamin E are primarily:

Vegetable oils

Nuts and seeds

Wheat germ

As you can see, antioxidants are a vital part of a healthy diet, and an important means of reducing your risk of osteoarthritis and rheumatoid arthritis. However, you cannot depend on antioxidants alone, so let's look at other nutrients that play a part in a healthy body.

Note! ➡
Recommended Daily Allowances established by the Food and Nutrition Board, National Academy of Sciences.

	Vit A mcg	Vit D mcg	Vit E mcg	Vit C mcg	Cal mg	Phosp mg	Mag mg
Infants							
0 to 6 months	375	7.5	3	30	400	300	40
6-12	375	10	4	35	600	500	60
Children							
1 to 3 years	400	10	6	40	800	800	80
4 to 6	500	10	7	45	800	800	120
7 to 10	700	10	7	45	800	800	170
Males							
11 to 14	1000	10	10	50	1200	1200	270
15 to 18	1000	10	10	60	1200	1200	400
19 to 24	1000	10	10	60	1200	1200	350
25 to 50	1000	5	10	60	800	800	350
51-plus	1000	5	10	60	800	800	350
Females							
11 to 14	800	10	8	50	1200	1200	280
15 to 18	800	10	8	60	1200	1200	300
19 to 24	800	10	8	60	1200	1200	280
25 to 50	800	5	8	60	800	800	280
51-plus	800	5	8	60	800	800	280
Pregnant/ Lactating							
1st 6 months	1300	10	12	95	1200	1200	355
2nd 6 months	1200	10	11	90	1200	1200	340

Calcium

At this moment, 98 percent of your body's calcium resides in your bones and the rest circulates in the blood, taking part in metabolic functions. Since your body cannot manufacture calcium, you must eat calcium-rich foods every day to replace what is lost. When your diet lacks sufficient calcium to replace the amount that has been excreted, your body begins to break down bone to retrieve the calcium it needs for life-preserving metabolic processes.

Consuming calcium-rich foods will help you meet your recommended daily requirements, but the calcium will not replace any calcium that is already gone. As we mentioned before, absorbing calcium from your digestive tract also requires the presence of vitamin D. Ten to 15 minutes of exposure to the sun will help your body to manufacture vitamin D. Absorbing calcium for bone health also requires magnesium and phosphorus.

Calcium can be found in:

Milk and milk products

Carrot juice

Soy and soy products

Sesame and sunflower seeds

Yogurt

Ricotta

Cheese

Oysters

Salmon

Collard greens

Spinach

Bright Idea
For those who cannot tolerate dairy products, calcium is also found in seafood, such as salmon and oysters, spinach, broccoli, and oranges. You can also take a calcium supplement, preferably with a meal, to help absorb the calcium from the stomach. Ask your physician before taking any supplements.

Ice cream

Cottage cheese

Kale

Broccoli

Oranges

Magnesium and phosphorus

Magnesium and phosphorus are minerals that help calcium to do its job. Magnesium can be found in leafy green vegetables, nuts, soybeans, seeds, and whole grains. Phosphorus is good for the bones, but too much can actually increase your need for more calcium. Phosphorus is found in many processed foods and soft drinks.

Fluoride

Although fluoride is generally associated with toothpaste and healthy teeth, fluoride is just as important for strengthening bones. Studies have shown that communities with fluoridated water have reported less incidences of osteoporosis, although fluoride is not an FDA-approved method of treating or preventing osteoporosis. Sources of fluoride include fish, tea, and most animal foods.

Guess what helps my pain?

Your friend, who suffers from rheumatoid arthritis, might claim that eating a little bit of fish every day helps to keep his symptoms at bay. A co-worker might vow that eliminating red peppers from her diet has helped to eliminate her morning stiffness. Is there something behind this? Can you believe that one particular food helped to reduce their symptoms?

The medical community has not proven any of these claims, but some foods have been shown to decrease the inflammation in your joints. It definitely is not a cure for arthritis, but it is a start. Now we will examine the various foods that patients have claimed helped reduce their symptoms.

Omega-3 fatty acids

Omega-3 fatty acids have already been touted as a way to decrease the risk of coronary heart disease. Now researchers believe that omega-3 fatty acids may have an anti-inflammatory effect. Studies have shown that patients with rheumatoid arthritis who have taken omega-3 fatty acids, in supplement form, experienced significant reduction in pain and swelling, and an improvement in morning stiffness and fatigue.

Research is still being conducted to see if omega-3 fatty acids can be an alternative to non-steroidal anti-inflammatory drugs, the drugs that fight inflammation of arthritis.

It has also been shown that omega-3 fatty acids decrease the production of tumor necrosis factor (TNF), a protein produced in high levels of chronic illness, such as rheumatoid arthritis patients.

However, the American Dietetic Association states that fish oil supplements that contain omega-3 fatty acids are not recommended as a substitute for fish, or as a dietary supplement. Omega-3 fatty acids can be found in seafood, especially higher-fat fish, such as albacore tuna, mackerel, and salmon, or it can be taken as a dietary supplement.

The side effects of omega-3 fatty acids are minimal, consisting largely of nausea, flatulence, and diarrhea.

Nightshade foods

Foods such as tomatoes, potatoes, eggplant, peppers, and chilies have been dubbed the "nightshade" family. It is believed that the solanine—an alkaloid found in these foods—causes morning stiff-ness. Medical studies have not shown any connection between nightshade foods and arthritis, but believers have eliminated these foods from their diet.

Oh soy!

New research suggests that soy foods, like tofu or soymilk, may be vital for preserving bones. A study of postmenopausal women who consumed foods rich in soy's isoflavones found that eating soy restored some of the calcium in the women's bones. The study measured bone density at the lumbar spine, a part of the body at the small of the back that is vulnerable to fractures due to osteoporosis. Since the medical community is uncertain that calcium that has been lost can be replaced, more research on soy needs to be completed.

Eliminating purines

Purines are the end products of the digestion of proteins. Some purines are made in the body, but some are in drugs and substances including caffeine. People who have a problem eliminating purines from the body may suffer from gout. A low-purine diet or a purine-free diet may be necessary. Foods that are high in purines include anchovies, sardines, liver, kidneys, organ meats, legumes, and poultry. The foods with the lowest purine levels include vegetables other than legumes, eggs, fruit, cheese, nuts, sugar, and gelatin.

Dietary supplements

No one food contains all of the vitamins that you need, and with few exceptions, vitamins cannot be made in the body. As a result, you may need to take vitamin supplements in order to obtain the necessary nutrients to remain healthy.

Even though these products are sold over-the-counter, they may not provide the benefits they claim. Others may have harmful side effects, especially when combined with particular foods or prescription medications. It is important to discuss dietary supplements with a registered dietitian and your pharmacist.

Before you start popping supplements:

- Make sure you are eating enough. If you are not consuming enough food each day, a supplement will help you meet your requirements. However, food is necessary for energy and other means of sustaining a healthy body.

- Talk with your physician and pharmacist. Make sure they know exactly what supplements you are taking, how much and how often, and what other medications you are currently taking. This will eliminate any possible dangerous interactions with other drugs you may be taking.

- Do not exceed the dosage your physician has recommended to you.

- Don't overdo it. If you believe in the "If a little is good, more is better" philosophy, you might suffer from dangerous side effects when you take vitamins in large doses. For example, as we mentioned earlier, too much vitamin C can trigger rheumatoid arthritis or cancer. This also applies when taken in a supplement form.

Chondroitin sulfate and glucosamine

There are some claims that nutritional supplements can relieve the pain of osteoarthritis and even regenerate the deteriorating cartilage in the joints. A few years ago, Dr. Jason Theodosakis authored the book *The Miracle Cure*. This book caused quite a stir

Unofficially... The National Institutes of Health (NIH) has launched an Internet database of accumulated scientific studies on dietary supplements. The database contains 250,000 citations from more than 3,000 journals. IBIDS can be accessed through the Office of Dietary Supplements' web site (http://dietary-supplements.info.nih.gov) and the USDA's web site (http://www.nal.usda.gov/fnic/IBIDS).

in the medical community when Dr. Theodosakis stated that the combination of two nutritional supplements, chondroitin sulfate and glucosamine, can relieve the pain of osteoarthritis, halt, reverse and even cure osteoarthritis, and regenerate deteriorating cartilage in joints.

According to Theodosakis, these supplements pass through the blood to the joints, where they stimulate the production of new cartilage cells and reduce the action of enzymes that harm cartilage. Sales of these dietary supplements soon skyrocketed, but medical experts do not necessarily support the claims made in the book.

Glucosamine is a substance that is synthesized by the body and can play a role in repairing cartilage. It is believed that it may stimulate cartilage cell growth and may inhibit the enzymes that break down this process.

Chondroitin, is also naturally found in cartilage, and the author claims that it can also stop the enzymes that break down the cartilage. Combining these two substances together, the author claims, boosts the actions of the other.

However, according to the American Academy of Orthopaedic Surgeons, little evidence exists to show that these products relieve chronic joint pain. The American College of Rheumatology and the Arthritis Foundation also do not recommend these dietary supplements as preventative measures of osteoarthritis. All of these organizations have publicly stated that further studies are needed before any formal support of the product can be made.

Food and medication

You probably know that it is potentially dangerous to mix two different medications because of the possible side effects, but did you know that it might be just as dangerous to mix your medications with certain foods, dietary supplements, or herbal supplements? Did you also know that your medications might effect the benefits of the foods you are eating? For example, corticosteroids, prescribed for rheumatoid arthritis and ulcerative colitis, can decrease calcium absorption and cause an increase of calcium in the urine. Methotrexate and sulfasalazine can interfere with the benefits of folic acid, a B vitamin that is needed for cell growth. Your doctor will probably supplement your medications with the crucial vitamin that may be affected. It is important to take your medication as directed.

- Some medication needs to be taken with food. For example, nonsteroidal anti-inflammatory drugs (NSAIDs) can irritate the lining of the stomach and need to be taken with food to prevent any gastrointestinal irritation.

- Some medications need to be taken on an empty stomach.

- Some medications and food cannot be consumed within a certain time period of each other.

- Some medications need to be taken with plenty of water. Again, NSAIDs are best taken with at least 8 ounces of water to prevent gastrointestinal irritation.

- No medication should ever be mixed with alcohol.

It is important to read the directions on the bottle and to ask the pharmacist about any special instructions or interactions with foods.

Moneysaver
It is impossible to list all of the medications and foods that cause potential side effects when combined. Send for a copy of the brochure "Food & Drug Interactions," published by the National Consumer League (NCL). Visit their web site at www.nclnet.org, or send $2 to NCL, 1701 K Street NW, Suite 1200, Washington, DC, 20006.

Bright Idea
If you believe you have a food allergy, start a food diary and list all the foods you eat. Compare the food diary to your symptom diary and see if exposure to certain foods trigger or worsen your symptoms.

Food allergies

Some patients with arthritis have stated that certain foods may trigger or exasperate their arthritis symptoms. A food allergy means that a specific food has caused an inflammatory response, which can include hives, facial swelling, and anaphylactic shock (a severe and possibly fatal allergic response).

Again, except for gout, there is no medical evidence that links one particular food to an increase in arthritis symptoms. However, if you believe that one particular food is bothering your arthritis symptoms, try to eliminate that food from your diet. If you do not know which food may be the trigger, try an elimination diet. An elimination diet pares your diet down to a few harmless foods. One at a time, you will slowly add back in the possible culprits until you notice any particular increase in symptoms. Keep a log of what you have done to show your physician.

Phytochemicals

You will probably hear more about phytochemicals in the next few years as researchers learn more about what these substances are and how they benefit your health.

The American Dietetic Association states that phytochemicals, "are substances that plants naturally produce to protect themselves against viruses, bacteria, and fungi. And they include hundreds of naturally occurring substances, including carotenoids, flavonoids, indoles, isoflavones, capsaicin, and protease inhibitors. Different plant foods supply different kinds and amounts of phytochemicals." These substances are in vegetables, legumes, fruits and whole grains. How the phytochemicals affect your health are still being researched.

Obesity

Studies have shown that obese people have an increased risk—up to five times greater to develop osteoarthritis—than people of average or below average weight. Recent studies also show that being overweight at a young age is associated with osteoarthritis of the knee in later life. Obesity has also been connected to gout. Losing excess weight is beneficial to your health. Unfortunately, many people do not know how to properly lose weight.

More often than not, people want to lose the weight quickly. So they try fad diets that claim that by eating one particular food for a week, you will lose 5 pounds. Of course you will. You have eliminated all the other healthy nutrients from your body. The bad news is that when you start eating properly again, you will gain back the weight that you lost. Then you will probably start another fad diet, believing that you have failed this one. It is a vicious cycle that you will start over and over again.

Put an end to that vicious cycle.

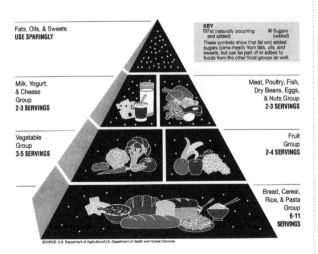

← Note!
USDA food pyramid

Unofficially...
Every year
Americans spend
more than $30
billion in the
weight-loss
industry, mostly
on fad diets and
lose-weight-quick
schemes.

Eating the right foods on a daily basis provides the energy you need to get through the day and perform physical activities. It also helps your body remain healthy and strong, and helps decrease your risk of illness.

The right foods will prevent dehydration and injury, and help quickly heal any injuries that might occur.

The number of calories you should consume each day depends on a few factors, including your age, metabolic rate (the rate that you burn calories), and body composition, or ratio of fat to muscle.

Just like it is important to have a basic knowledge of your body, you should also have a basic understanding of what your body needs to remain healthy. In addition to the vital nutrients we have already discussed—and some we haven't—your body also needs carbohydrates, fats, proteins, and water.

Carbohydrates

Carbohydrates are the body's main fuel source, and should comprise 55 to 65 percent of all the calories you take in each day. There are two types of carbohydrates:

- Simple, such as fruit, are absorbed more quickly into the bloodstream.

- Complex, including breads, cereals, potatoes, and pasta. Complex carbohydrates provide a steady stream of energy and are best eaten before a sustained workout.

You might have heard of carb, or carbo, loading. This is eating a large amount of carbohydrates. Only intense physical activity, such as a marathon, requires carbo-loading.

Fats and proteins

While carbohydrates are the body's primary source of fuel for exercise, fats will be converted into energy if you sustain an activity. In other words, if you are trying to lose weight, you will not burn off fat until all of the carbohydrates that you have stored have been depleted. When that happens, the body turns to the fat stores.

Less than 30 percent of your daily calories should come from fat, preferably unsaturated sources. Choose healthy foods that are low in saturated fat, such as avocados, olives, seeds, and nuts.

Protein is also called upon to provide energy when fat and carbohydrate stores are depleted. Unfortunately, the body must break down muscle to obtain energy from protein: Protein traditionally supplies amino acids, which are needed to build, maintain, and repair body tissues, including muscle. Individual protein needs vary depending on a person's activity level. A general recommendation is that 15 to 20 percent of your total daily calories should come from protein. Healthy, protein-rich foods include lean meats, fish, low-fat dairy, nuts, beans, and tofu.

Bright Idea
Consider your activity level when you are determining how many calories you need. The more active you are, the more food you need to eat.

Drink up!

Water is necessary for energy production, temperature control, digestion, and elimination of byproducts from the body. It also cushions the body's tissues and organs to protect them from any potential injuries. Water is especially vital for people who exercise regularly, as they are more likely to suffer from dehydration.

To properly hydrate the body, drink at least 16 oz. of water before and after your workout and 4 oz. every 15 minutes during the activity—even if you do not feel thirsty. Thirst is actually a symptom of dehydration.

Stick with pure spring water—sports drinks are often high in sugar and calories and meet the needs of only marathon runners and other endurance athletes. Avoid caffeinated beverages such as soda or iced tea.

Vegetarian diets

Studies have shown that people with rheumatoid arthritis may benefit from a vegetarian diet, but researchers are not exactly sure why. One school of thought is that meat affects the type of fatty acids in your blood and can affect inflammation. When rheumatoid arthritis patients eliminate meat from their diet, they are reducing the risk of inflammation. Vegetarian diets dramatically reduce the overall amount of fat in the diet, as well, adding another benefit of eliminating excess weight.

If you decide to follow a vegetarian plan and eliminate meat from your diet, make sure that you get enough protein from other sources. Protein is the main building material for muscles, blood, skin, hair, and nails. Vegetarian foods high in protein are soy-based foods, beans, nuts, eggs, milk, and cheese. Not enough protein in your diet causes weakness, depression, increased risk of infection, and slow recovery from disease.

Labeling foods

We have all seen the commercials where manufacturers of various products claim that their product can cure "this" or reduce your risk of "that." Now manufacturers have to watch what they say. In 1990, Congress passed the Nutrition Labeling and Education Act (NLEA). Food labels provide a reliable source of applicable nutrition information for consumers on a Nutrition Facts panel. In addition to the Nutrition Facts panel, products may use the FDA's pre-approved health claims, which are based on scientific evidence and agreement among specialists in the field of food and nutrition.

Children and diet

In Chapter one, we discussed how a bone grows and how, at birth, a newborn has more bones than an adult. As the child grows, cartilage is replaced by bone, and the bones fuse together to create larger units. Eventually, the skeleton has 206 adult bones, formed through a process called ossification. These bones continue to lengthen and harden until the child is about twenty years old, at which point the bones are considered fully developed.

Good nutrition helps the child to grow and develop healthy bones. Without it, bones may not grow properly.

Calcium is one of the most important nutrients in a child's diet. By eating well, children build up their bone mass and protect themselves against the later development of osteoporosis and the degeneration of their bones. Unfortunately, recent studies show that most children do not consume the appropriate daily requirement of calcium, a mineral that plays an essential role in creating bone mass. Children under 5 years are only getting about 46 percent of the recommended daily requirement of calcium.

Two or three servings of milk, a source of calcium, fill a child's daily requirement. Milk also includes vitamin D, which the body needs in order to absorb calcium and other vitamins and minerals. Other sources of calcium are green leafy vegetables, such as broccoli and kale; and fish, including salmon and sardines; tofu; kidney beans; almonds; and sesame seeds. Calcium-fortified foods—such as orange juice, bread, and cereal are also helpful.

Just the facts

- There are no miracle cures for arthritis.
- Antioxidants are beneficial to your health— remember colors when choosing foods rich in antioxidants.
- Eating right will help you to lose excess weight.
- Tell your doctor about any dietary supplements that you are taking to prevent any potential complications.
- If a manufacturer makes a claim that a product or food is too good to be true, it probably is.

Exercise and Arthritis

Chapter 13

I t is now a proven medical fact that physically active people are healthier and live longer that inactive people. A regular exercise program is beneficial for everyone, but exercise can especially help if you suffer from painful arthritis. Exercise reduces joint pain and stiffness and increases flexibility, muscle strength, and endurance. As a result, your daily activities will become easier to perform.

Sadly, however, studies claim that one-third of adults in the United States report no leisure-time physical activity. Even if you are an active person, you might find that your level of activity declines as your arthritic symptoms worsen. Although flare-ups can cause you to decrease your activity, leading a sedentary life is bad news for your joints. It can cause bones and joints to weaken over time. If you are carrying any extra pounds, it can further strain already stressed joints and muscles, cause tendons and ligaments to separate, and prevent joints from functioning properly. Regular exercise, combined with nutritious eating, can help you to reduce any excess weight you may be carrying and ease stress on your joints.

Watch Out!
Check with your doctor if you are middle-aged or older, or if you have not been physically active, before you begin any kind of exercise program. Ask your doctor if there are any kinds of exercises that are off-limits because of your particular type of arthritis.

Exercise is not just for the young and active. At any age, an exercise program is an essential component in slowing down the aging process and making your senior years more enjoyable. It is never too late to begin and maintain an exercise program.

Keep in mind, however, that exercise is only one part of a comprehensive arthritis treatment plan that can include many other methods of therapy. The National Institute of Arthritis and Musculoskeletal and Skin Diseases states (NIAMSD) that the amount and form of exercise recommended for each individual will vary depending on which arthritic joints are involved, the amount of inflammation, how stable the joints are, and whether you've had joint replacement surgery. Work with both a skilled physician and physical therapist who are knowledgeable about the medical and rehabilitation needs of people with arthritis, to design an exercise plan for you.

Do not rush into an exercise program or expect quick results. You might do more damage to your joints than good. Take your time and be patient and you will begin to see results.

Over the last decade, many studies have been done on the benefits of exercise for those suffering with arthritis. Based on these studies, three specific types of exercise have proven to be most beneficial to arthritis sufferers: range-of-motion, aerobic, and strengthening exercises.

This chapter will explain what these exercises are, how they can benefit your overall health, and specifically how exercising can help to ease your arthritis pain and strengthen your joints.

It will also help you to get started on an exercise program, learn how to maintain that motivation, and how to overcome any stumbling blocks along the way.

Types of exercises

Three types of exercises have been proven to help arthritis patients:

Range-of-motion exercises

Range-of-motion, or stretching, exercises help to maintain normal joint movement and to maintain or increase flexibility. These are gentle stretching exercises that help to move each joint as far as possible in all directions. These exercises need to be done daily to help keep joints fully mobile and prevent stiffness and deformities.

Aerobic or cardiovascular exercises

Aerobic means "with oxygen." To be considered aerobic, an activity must fit the following criteria: The exercise must be rhythmic, continuous, and involve the large muscles of the body; the heart and lungs need to work hard enough to provide the oxygen necessary for the increased work—that's the cardiovascular part; and the aerobic activity must be maintained for at least 15 to 20 minutes. For optimum benefits, aerobic exercise must be performed at least three times per week.

Aerobic exercise improves cardiovascular fitness and helps to burn calories and control weight. Weight control is important because excess weight puts pressure on your joints. Some studies show that aerobic exercise can also reduce inflammation in some joints.

Aerobic exercise also helps proper circulation of blood through the body. This is important to help get oxygen and nutrients to all the organs, tissues, and muscles, especially the heart. Aerobic exercise

Unofficially...
Billy Jean King, who won 20 Wimbledon titles, four U.S. Open singles championships and titles in both France and Australia, suffered from secondary osteoarthritis (resulting from injury). At 18, she slammed both knees into the dashboard during a car accident. Five years later she was diagnosed with osteoarthritis. King valued exercise as a vital component to rehabilitation.

helps to improve circulation because it strengthens vessels, increases blood supply, and decreases the risk of cardiovascular disease, which can narrow and weaken blood vessels. When muscles do not get an adequate supply of blood, they can cramp. Good blood circulation is also needed to help tissues heal after injuries.

Since aerobic exercise is defined as any activity that uses the large muscles of the body, is performed for at least 20 minutes, and works the heart within its target range, many activities can be considered aerobic.

The choices range from individual activities such as walking, running, cycling, rowing, or stair-climbing to group exercises, including aerobic dance, step-aerobics, and circuit training. More recent trends incorporate boxing and martial arts movements into an aerobic routine. Cultural trends have also spawned jazz and hip-hop aerobics.

Combining different aerobic activities is a good way to prevent boredom. Try performing a variety of exercises, such as running, cycling, and stair-climbing for a total of three sessions per week.

Unfortunately, for some arthritis patients, even a simple walk can be uncomfortable, and rowing, cycling, or stair climbing are simply out of the question. If this is how you feel, do not give up. Instead, hit the water!

When you are in water, your body is buoyant and there is no impact or pressure on your bones and joints. Moving in the water can be done without pain. The water also reduces the amount of stiffness in the joint. Water exercises (also called hydrotherapy) are not an easy workout. Your body actually works harder to get through the water, which provides good strength-training benefits.

If you can join a gym or local Y, water exercises are a good alternative when the weather turns on you. Here are a few examples of water exercises:

- Walk through the water while moving your arms in a swim stroke motion.

- Alternate walking with swimming laps.

- Move your arms and legs as if you were skipping rope.

- Go backward and forward.

Strengthening exercises

Strength refers to the maximum force that can be generated by a specific muscle or muscle group. The more strength muscles have, the more they can lift. This does not mean that you need large muscles to be strong. While some muscles or groups of muscles may be stronger than others, overall strength is important. It enhances the ability to perform activities, such as carrying baskets of laundry, and taking care of the lawn and garden.

Until recently, aerobic exercise was the only training routine recommended for optimal health benefits. Today, strength training, also known as resistance training, is recognized as an integral part of overall fitness.

Research has also shown a direct relationship with simple strength exercises of the quadriceps (thigh muscles) and the reduction of knee pain and disability associated with osteoarthritis. Significant decreases in pain, and improvements in physical function and strength of the quadriceps, were found in those who enrolled in an exercising program.

In 1996, a Tufts University study found that even people with severe rheumatoid arthritis could safely

Bright Idea
Whether or not you are an experienced swimmer, make sure there is a lifeguard on duty wherever you perform your water exercises. Never exercise alone. Fatigue or muscle cramps can make it difficult to get out of the water without help. This can put your life in jeopardy.

increase their strength by roughly 60 percent in 12 weeks through a modest weight-training program. They were careful not to exercise during flare-ups and to rest whenever they felt joint pain, returning to strength training once a flare-up had passed.

You can increase your strength by performing resistance exercises that challenge your muscles. Increasing your strength is not the same as muscular endurance, however. Muscular endurance refers to the ability of a muscle to perform multiple repetitions of an exercise before the muscle is fatigued. Minimal force and resistance are used when training to achieve muscular endurance.

Women are often afraid of resistance training fearing they will bulk up with muscle. However, large quantities of testosterone are needed to gain massive muscle size—women just do not have enough. They will gain only strength and some muscle definition.

Different forms of resistance training include:

- Free weights and machines.

- Isometrics (pitting one muscle against another).

- Elastic bands.

- Sstep straps.

- Using your own or a partner's weight against your own body weight.

When you start strengthening exercises, start with your own resistance or one- or two-pound weights and progress slowly. Beginners will obtain maximum benefits progressing from easy to more difficult exercises. The general recommendation for the beginner is to work the larger muscles (back, chest, legs) before the smaller muscle groups (biceps, triceps, shoulders, calves). This sequence

Watch Out!
When performing strength exercises, correct positioning is crucial. Doing exercises incorrectly can cause muscle tears and more pain and swelling.

fatigues the larger muscles early in the workout when the energy is high.

Maintaining adequate strength is an important concern with advancing age. Without regular strength training, muscles become weak. As you age, you lose a total of 10 to 12 percent of your strength, particularly between the ages of 30 and 65. This can result in a decreased activity level, possible injury to your muscles and bones, and an increased risk of bone disease and conditions, such as osteoporosis and arthritis.

On your mark...starting an exercise program

Now you know the different types of beneficial exercises to do for your arthritis, but how do you get started? The American Heart Association suggests keeping several factors in mind when choosing an exercise program:

- Your health and physical capabilities.

- Your interests (whether you prefer group or individual exercises).

- Proficiency and adaptability; do not be discouraged if you are a little clumsy initially.

- Necessary equipment and facilities for a particular exercise or sport.

- Seasonal adaptability (varying activities according to the weather).

- Scheduling 30 to 60 minute sessions, three to four times per week.

- The kind of exercise you choose should be fun and demanding, but not exhausting.

- What your doctor wants you to do.

Unofficially...
Studies show that it takes two to three weeks to improve from your beginning fitness level; six weeks to three months to achieve significant improvement; and three to six months to achieve maximum fitness results. Once you have started your exercise program, reassess your progress every three months. Revise your workout routine to reflect your progress to date and assist you in reaching your new fitness goals.

How long should you work out?

Current recommendations are for 30 minutes of moderate activity on most days of the week, or three 10-minute sessions throughout the course of the day.

Keep in mind, however, that while this is the recommendation, it does not mean that you can perform 30 minutes of exercise on your first attempt. Take it slow. If you walk for only a few minutes the first day, do not get discouraged. The benefits of an exercise program will show up when you maintain the program on a regular basis. You should see small results along the way. Perhaps the next week, increase your walk to 10 minutes, and the next month you might try 20 minutes. Do not expect too much or you will be disappointed.

Too much too soon?

Did you overdo it at the gym the first time out and your muscles seem to be paying you back? Over-exercising is using your body too hard for too long a time. A regular exercise program provides many benefits, and it is normal to be mildly sore and a little tired following your workouts. You might even push yourself beyond your limits at times, and that is okay too. But if you overdo it without allowing your body to recover, your body can break down.

The signs of doing too much include:

- Unusual or persistent fatigue.
- Increased weakness.
- Decreased range of motion.
- Increased joint swelling.
- Continuing pain that lasts beyond an hour or so after exercising.

Bright Idea
The right sneakers are a vital part of a proper exercise program. Do not sacrifice for a cheaper pair. Shop in the evening when your feet are swollen. Wear socks and try on more than one size of the same shoe to ensure proper fit. Leave a finger-width space between your longest toe and the shoe tip. Remember: the best footwear does not need much "breaking in."

The tips below will help keep your body healthy so you can exercise safely:

- Practice patience. If you think that over-exercising will lead to faster results, you are wrong.

- Cut down on your current routine or choose easier exercises until your body has time to recover.

- Take at least one day off between workouts and get plenty of sleep.

If a joint is stretched beyond its normal range of motion, it is said to be sprained; an overextended muscle or ligament is said to be strained. Joints that are repeatedly injured can eventually weaken, so it is vital to allow a full recovery, provide proper treatment, and learn important prevention techniques. Here are the basic principles of safe exercise to keep in mind:

- **Awareness:** Pay attention to your body's messages. If you feel pain, stop working out or modify the activity immediately.

- **Environment:** Dress for the weather when planning for your workout. Stiff, cold joints are prone to injury.

- **Training:** No matter what the activity, learn to do it with proper technique.

- **Warm up/cool down:** Slowly ease your body into and out of a workout.

- **Stretching:** Increases blood flow to your muscles before working out.

- **Shoes:** Sport-specific shoes help prevent pressure on the joints.

Treat it: RICE

If you sprain or strain a joint or muscle, treat the injury promptly with "RICE." In the exercise world, "RICE" stands for:

- **Rest:** Reduce or discontinue the activity immediately.

- **Ice:** Apply an ice pack immediately to decrease swelling and blood flow to the injured area. If swelling continues, apply the pack for no more than 10 minutes at a time, then wait 10 more before reapplying. Continue until swelling subsides.

- **Compression:** To restrict movement and reduce swelling, wrap the injured area firmly in an elastic bandage, but not too tight—it can cut off circulation.

- **Elevation:** The injury should be elevated higher than the heart until swelling goes down. This will prevent excess fluids and blood from building up in the area.

Some injuries cannot be treated at home and may require a doctor's consultation. For example, the application of ice on a swollen joint causes vasoconstriction in Raynaud's patients, which may trigger a painful episode.

Get out of the gym

Exercising does not mean confinement to a health club. There are many different styles of exercise that also benefit arthritis patients, from yoga to gardening to martial arts.

Yoga and you

The word "yoga" literally means union. It is an ancient Hindu mind-body technique that promotes physical, mental, and emotional harmony. Through

Watch Out!
Consult your physician immediately if you suspect a traumatic injury, the pain does not subside, there is pain in the joint after two weeks, or if you have a sign of infection. Use your intuition. If you feel like something might be wrong, get examined by a physician.

a series of poses accompanied by deep breathing and concentration skills, yoga calms the mind and spirit while allowing the body to become more limber. Breathing deeply and rhythmically may slow the heart beat, lower blood pressure, and decrease the release of tension-causing adrenaline. Many health clubs and community centers offer this antidote to unwinding.

Martial arts makes for stronger bones

The many forms of martial arts are not only practiced for self-defense purposes, but are also used for exercise, relaxation, and spirituality. Because martial arts involve the entire body, they increase muscular strength, enhance balance and agility, develop flexibility, and improve cardiovascular fitness. These techniques also require intense concentration and the ability to relax and focus. As a result, practicing martial arts can help decrease stress levels and improve concentration.

To obtain the maximum physical and mental benefits from martial arts, attend classes at least twice a week. The length and intensity of each class will vary, depending on the students' abilities and the style of martial art. Generally, though, martial arts classes last about an hour and incorporate both stretching and traditional self-defense moves.

T'ai Chi Ch'aun—it really works!

T'ai Chi Ch'aun, also called t'ai chi, is a gentle form of exercise that provides a good introduction to martial arts. It includes slow, nonstop, circular movements, which help people control their body and learn proper breathing techniques.

T'ai chi's self-paced exercises are terrific for individuals at any fitness level. The slowness of the

Watch Out!
Many forms of martial arts, such as karate, judo, and aikido, require the ability to withstand throws and blows to the body. They are not recommended for older people or beginners. Novices should choose a soft-fist or noncontact style, such as t'ai chi ch'aun, as an introduction.

Bright Idea
Selecting a form of martial arts depends on your interest in individual or group training, desire for competitive versus non-competitive exercise, and your physical abilities. Every class is progressive: Your level of fitness will increase as you train. Observe a class before joining. Classes are held in studios called dojos or do-jangs, and can be found at a local Y or community center.

movements and the circular actions involved, however, can make t'ai chi difficult to learn.

T'ai chi should be practiced on a regular basis. Studies show that regular t'ai chi practice, at least three times a week, reduces tension levels, depression, and anxiety while increasing energy. T'ai chi exercise also improves balance and coordination, strengthens major muscle groups, and reinforces proper posture.

Get fit gardening

Gardening is a fun hobby for many, and it is also a terrific workout that uses all the major muscle groups of the body. You can burn as much fat weeding and shoveling as you can riding a bicycle.

Studies have shown that gardening activities such as shoveling, hoeing, raking, and weeding strengthen muscles, burn calories, and increase flexibility. In addition, gardening decreases stress hormones and lowers blood pressure. So, when you are pruning the bushes or mowing the lawn, you are probably getting a healthy dose of exercise.

Back injuries and joint pain from repetitive activities are common in gardeners who dig, lift heavy compost bags, rake leaves, or hoe. Improper lifting, twisting, and stretching are the main causes of these injuries. You can prevent gardening injuries and increased joint pain by:

- Using ergonomically designed gardening tools and those with long handles. These are specially designed tools that set handles at the correct angle to prevent pressure to the wrist and reduce the risk of carpal tunnel syndrome.

- Use a four-wheeled cart. Throwing bags over your shoulder or using a wheelbarrow can cause improper distribution of weight on your back. Wheelbarrows are not even recommended anymore.

- Do not twist your spine when working in the garden. Instead, face the same direction as your shovel and insert it vertically to provide the most leverage.

Exercise and breathing

Breathing is a necessary function that most people never have to think about, but proper breathing is an important aspect of exercise: It provides energy-giving oxygen, eliminates carbon dioxide from the body, and maximizes the benefits of a workout.

With proper breathing during exercises, muscles, especially the heart, will receive an adequate amount of oxygen and blood. Breathing improperly, such as holding your breath or breathing too fast, can cause dizziness or shortness of breath.

There are different styles of breathing for different activities. Stretching utilizes slower, deeper breathing that is held and released during different parts of the stretch. In weight training, it is vital not to hold your breath, but to inhale and exhale throughout the routine. Aerobic exercise does not have a formal breathing pattern, but the ability to speak comfortably during a workout signifies correct breathing.

Exercise and nutrition

Exercise and proper eating go hand in hand. Good nutrition fuels exercise and, in turn, exercise boosts metabolism, causing the body to burn extra calories during and after a workout.

Eating the right foods provides the energy needed to get through a workout as well as perform

Bright Idea
If you like hiking or climbing, but are afraid about the abuse your joints might take, consider using a walking stick. Walking sticks can help your body absorb much of your lower body weight, but must be used correctly. This leads to considerable spine and joint relief, especially when you have pre-existing joint and spinal diseases, such as arthritis, or spondylitis.

activities of everyday living. Physical activity places a demand on the body. As a result, you use energy, lose bodily fluids, and put stress on the muscles, joints, and bones. The right foods will reenergize you, prevent dehydration and injury, and help to quickly heal any injuries that might occur.

The number of calories you should consume each day depends on your fitness program:

- How long you exercise (duration).

- How often you exercise (frequency).

- The intensity of the exercise.

Your calorie needs will also depend on your age, basic metabolic rate, and body composition, or ratio of fat to muscle. The more you exercise, the more food you need to provide energy.

Watch your water intake

Water is necessary for all energy production in the body, temperature control, and the elimination of by-products from the body. It also cushions the body's tissues and organs to protect them from any potential injuries. Water is especially vital for regular exercisers, as they are more susceptible to mild dehydration.

To properly hydrate the body, drink at least 16 ounces of water before and after your workout and four ounces every 15 minutes during the activity—even if you do not feel thirsty. Thirst is actually a symptom of dehydration. But to relieve that thirst, it's best to stick with water—sports drinks are often high in sugar and calories and really only meet the needs of marathon runners or endurance athletes.

Carbohydrate consciousness

There are two types of carbohydrates, simple and complex. Simple carbohydrates, such as fruits, are

Watch Out!
If you like to consume a hearty dinner, you might be sabotaging your weight-management efforts. Studies show that you burn 75 percent of your calories within the first 12 hours after you wake up, typically 7 a.m. to 7 p.m. Only 25 percent of your daily calories will be burned later than evening. Eat a hearty breakfast instead of a big dinner and plan your exercise program early in the day to maximize caloric expenditure.

sugars; complex carbohydrates include bread, cereals, and pasta. Both supply energy for exercise, but simple carbohydrates are absorbed more quickly into the bloodstream. Complex carbohydrates provide a steady stream of energy and are better for a more sustained workout.

Carbohydrates should comprise about 55 to 65 percent of your total daily caloric intake. Only intense physical activity, such as a marathon, require carbo-loading, or eating lots of carbohydrates before an event.

Fats and proteins: fuel for fitness

While carbohydrates are the primary fuel, fats and proteins will be converted into energy if the activity is sustained. For exercise to be fat-burning, it must be maintained and carbohydrate stores depleted. Regular, sustained exercise helps utilize fat stores.

Protein is also called upon to provide energy when fats and carbohydrates are in short supply. Unfortunately, the body must break down muscle to obtain energy from protein. Protein traditionally supplies amino acids, the building blocks needed to build, maintain, and repair body tissues.

Healthy protein-rich foods include lean meats, fish, low-fat dairy, nuts, beans, and tofu.

Kids and exercise

Exercise boosts the energy of children to meet the demands of their growing bodies. It also helps them build endurance, strength, and flexibility. Not only does exercise promote good health, it can also decrease a child's risk of illness. It is the most natural way to combat childhood obesity and high cholesterol levels, both more common in today's fast-food and video lifestyle. In addition, exercise

Bright Idea
Inactivity speeds the loss of calcium, which is needed for bone strength and muscle contraction. Increase your intake of calcium and vitamin D, which is needed for calcium absorption, by eating foods rich in these nutrients, such as cheese, eggs, some fish (sardines and salmon) and fortified cereals. Foods containing zinc may be helpful in boosting immunity and in healing bone fractures. Zinc-rich foods include meat, eggs, seafood, poultry, milk, and whole grains.

can positively contribute to your child's self-esteem. And strong, healthy children often perform better, both physically and academically.

Children need daily activity year-round, so it's never too early to instill a positive, healthy attitude toward exercise. How do you know if your child is getting enough exercise? The American Academy of Pediatrics has no physical requirements for ages six and under; they usually get enough exercise just doing "kid stuff." But older children need specific amounts of aerobic, stretching, and muscle-conditioning activities.

Experts warn, however, that intense, long-term training that includes rhythmic bouncing, such as jogging, can take its toll on your child's joints. Also, youngsters who are eager to begin weight training should seek proper guidance to prevent injury to growing muscles.

Children with the two most common forms of juvenile arthritis, juvenile ankylosing spondylitis (which inflames the spine), and juvenile rheumatoid arthritis (which makes joints hurt, swell, and stiffen), need to exercise just as much as any other children do—but the discomfort of the joints and spine can make it difficult to institute a regular exercise regimen for them. So special care must be taken to find the right exercise program—one that they will keep at regularly. Almost all options of exercise for adults are available for children, including:

- **Swimming:** creates virtually no strain on the joints.

- **Bicycling:** also good for the lower body. A stationary bicycle works just as well, especially in the cold weather when your child might be stuck inside for the weather.

> **"**
> My children will always run around when they have friends over, so I let them invite some friends over and have a backyard exercise olympics. To make it more fun, you can give out medals to everyone, but do not focus on winning.
> —Lisa, 33
> **"**

And remember, hand exercises are important to prevent muscle atrophy or weakness. If a child is bored or reluctant to exercise, she might need a little motivation. Start by setting an example at home:

- Plan outings to zoos, parks, and fairs that make walking necessary. Finish with a nutritious picnic.

- Limit television viewing. Children will naturally find ways to play if television is not an option.

- When the weather is bad, put on music and dance or rent a kids' exercise video.

- Choose active vacations. Go hiking, camping, or skiing. Involve the children in the decision-making process—they will be more inspired to participate.

- Local activity centers are terrific for rainy-day fun and for active, game-filled birthday parties.

Clothing and exercise

Looking good while you exercise is important to many individuals, especially if you are working out in a health club. But exercise clothes should be functional, as well as fashionable. The right apparel will:

- Protect you from harsh weather.

- Allow freedom of movement.

- Permit your pores to breath.

Different sports call for different clothes. You will also dress based on whether you are inside or outside, it is day or night, or in hot or cold weather.

The questions you should ask yourself when searching for exercise apparel are:

- Will your movements be hampered?

Moneysaver
Before buying cloths, try them on. Move around in the outfit; look in a mirror to see how the garment fits. Consider the nature of the activity you'll be performing: Twist, turn, squat, and bend over, checking every angle of movement. Close-fitting clothes should not pull or ride up. Pay attention to shoulder straps, crotch, backside, and legs. And keep your receipt.

- Are your clothes supporting your muscles and keeping them warm?

- Are your clothes keeping you comfortable and dry?

There are many issues to consider when buying sports apparel: fabric, fit/size, and durability.

Motivation

Motivation is the most important factor in a success-ful fitness program. Without it, you may lose the desire to work out and, as a result, become an exercise dropout. It is also difficult for you to stay motivated on the days that you have arthritis flare-ups.

Motivation is the inner drive that encourages you to work out on a regular basis. Maintaining this inner drive may take a little creativity. There are many physical and psychological benefits to becoming motivated. The physical benefits are obvious: you will exercise more regularly. Mentally, being successful with your workouts—in itself a great motivator—can boost your self-esteem.

Accept that you might slack off from time to time, but do not let a sidestep discourage you. Keep a list of your positive motivators and refer to it to get back on track. These suggestions will make exercise appealing and fun! Some motivational ideas include:

- Select exercise activities that will maintain your long-term interest. Change your workout routine every six to eight weeks to stave off boredom. Stay motivated by scheduling exercise appointments with yourself and setting small, more attainable goals.

- Pick a Partner! A workout partner counts on you to be ready for your workout. Your

Watch Out!
Exercising during the winter can be done safely, but only if the weather permits. Watch the temperature and wind-chill factors. Exercising in extreme cold temperatures or against high-speed winds can lead to serious conditions, such as hypothermia, when body temperature drops below 95°, or frostbite, when the skin freezes and skin cells are damaged. Find an alternative indoor activity.

commitment to a fitness plan then becomes vital to someone other than yourself. Partners share disappointments and achievements, and create fun and exciting ways to work out. Choose someone who enjoys the same things you do and who is at the same fitness level.

- Crank up the stereo! Studies show that people who read or watch television when they work out actually perform with less power and intensity because the distraction slows down their exercise pace. Instead, music has been found to stimulate the feel good chemicals of the brain, the "endorphins."

- Reward yourself! Developing a reward system is a great motivating tool when it comes to exercise, but eliminate food from the list of rewards. Using food as a reward defeats the purpose of a regular exercise program. Instead, treat yourself to a facial or massage. Or create an exercise account and stash away some cash for an outfit that flatters your newly toned figured.

Who's teaching you?

Whether you join a group fitness class or are exercising at home with a video, finding a qualified instructor is important. A top-notch instructor:

- Is certified by a national aerobics organization and regularly receives continuing education credits.

- Instructs the class rather than performs.

- Understands that not all participants will be at the same level of fitness.

- Demonstrates and modifies exercises for each fitness level.

Moneysaver
If you can not afford a membership to an exercise club, consider renting an exercise video before buying one, or investing in a computer software program that offers additional assistance in developing goals, fitness profiles, and charting progress. Many also offer nutritional analyses and motivational tips. Keep brief notes of your daily food intake and exercise activities and transfer them to your laptop or home computer daily.

- Motivates participants to enjoy the exercising—and to continue exercising.

Developed by the Arthritis Foundation in 1987 and revised in 1993, People with Arthritis Who Can Exercise (PACE) is a community-based group recreational exercise program offering both basic and advanced levels. The program has 72 exercises from which instructors can select. Exercises are performed sitting, standing, or on the floor. Also included are a variety of endurance-building activities, games, relaxation techniques, and health education topics. For more information contact PACE Catalog Center, Arthritis Foundation, PO Box 9020, Pittsfield, MA 01202-9945; (800) PACE-236 (722-3236).

Just the facts

- Before you begin your physical fitness program, it is important to have a medical evaluation and a fitness assessment done to determine your level of exercise.

- Start an exercise program slowly.

- Children can become easily frustrated. Consider your child's age, stage of development, and interest when selecting appropriate activities.

- Exercise should be fun, not a chore. Reward yourself when you achieve even the smallest results.

One Step Beyond

PART V

GET THE SCOOP ON...
Self-managing your arthritis ▪ Making your
house accessible ▪ Coping at work ▪ Sex
and arthritis ▪ Arthritis and your family ▪
Your legal rights

Living Well
with Arthritis

The comedian George Burns once said, "I get a standing ovation just from standing." While this vaudevillian cracked jokes about his century-old body to amuse his audiences, anyone who suffers from arthritis may empathize with the quips. After all, arthritis sufferers know it is not easy living with this chronic and often disabling condition. On some days you rightly deserve praise just for getting around.

Arthritis is not a convenient disease. Unexpected and inconvenient flare-ups can interrupt daily routines. Simple tasks that were once taken for granted, such as opening a jar, gripping soap, or using a knife, can become painfully difficult.

Chronic pain and fatigue will change your own life, but you may not realize that your condition can uproot your family's lives as well. Relatives must also adjust to the limitations of your arthritis. For example, children may miss the mother who was once active and vibrant, but is now crippled with the pain

of rheumatoid arthritis and can no longer participate in family hikes. Relationships are strained when
one partner may avoid lovemaking because it is too
painful or too tiring.

Arthritis can also affect your job. If your arthritis
is severe and interferes with your ability to do your
job, you may need to take a disability leave. Just envi-
sion a computer data operator who has rheumatoid
arthritis and can no longer input the information
without a daily struggle with pain. How does she
keep doing her job?

Fortunately, however, arthritis does not have to
strip you of your independence or completely crip-
ple your lifestyle. Living well with arthritis is more
than just remembering to take your daily dose of
painkillers or make appointments with your physicians. It means making lifestyle adjustments and
accepting help when you need it. This chapter will
show you the many ways of managing your disease,
including handy arthritis aids to help you with daily
tasks, and legal and employment resources to help
you to find a job or protect the one you already
have.

> **❝**
> Realizing that I
> will have
> rheumatoid
> arthritis for the
> rest of my life
> (as devastating
> as it may sound)
> is really the first
> step in living
> with it.
> —Kelly, 26
> **❞**

Self-management

Remember how we discussed your medical team in
an earlier chapter? The most important member of
that medical team is *you*. The medical community
recognizes the importance of your active participa-
tion in your care and is now advocating a policy of
self-management so you can have some control over
your treatment.

One such program was developed by The
Multipurpose Arthritis and Musculoskeletal Diseases
Center at Stanford University, supported by the
National Institute of Arthritis and Musculoskeletal

and Skin Diseases (NIAMSD). The Arthritis Self-Help Course teaches people with arthritis how to take a more active part in their arthritis care. The Arthritis Self-Help Course is taught by the Arthritis Foundation and consists of a 12- to 15-hour program that includes lectures on osteoarthritis, rheumatoid arthritis, exercise, pain management, medication, doctor-patient relationships, and nontraditional treatment. Check with your local Arthritis Foundation office for more information on classes in your area.

Although a course such as this is a good idea, and learning the skills is important in managing your disease, it might not be feasible for someone to attend such a program. Therefore, it is important to learn these skills through other means, such as books and support groups. Most important, the process of learning coping skills is mostly trial-and-error as you discover what techniques work for you.

Coping at home

Your home is supposed to be a safe haven, but when you have arthritis, it can become a hell. Climbing the stairs, dressing, and reaching for boxes in the pantry can trigger arthritis pain. How can you cope at home without packing it all in and moving?

Handy arthritis aids

Sometimes it is the little gadget that can make all the difference in your day. For example, there are bathtub grab bars, elevated toilet seats, knob turners, and extenders to help you reach out-of-the-way items or drive-through banking slots. These assistive devices can help you with the tasks and challenges of living at home, such as opening doors, bathing, dressing, cooking, and more.

Unofficially...
Men should tough it out and deal with pain, right? A study shows that men think so. As a result, men are not using strategies to help them handle pain. An Ohio State University study suggests that women use coping strategies such as relaxation more than men do. It also shows that women are better at decreasing the emotional impact of the severe pain on their lives.

These devices are not just for the frail, older segment of the population. Anyone who needs to alleviate joint stress from undue bending, stretching, and straining can reap the benefits of these devices. They can also help you to conserve energy and maintain your independence.

Wheelchairs and scooters

No one wants to admit that they need help getting around, but it might be necessary at some point. How can you determine if it is time for you to use a walker, wheelchair, or scooter? Do you:

- Have difficulty lifting your legs?

- Find it hard to sit down then get back up again?

- Find it difficult to walk long distances without pain?

If you need a wheelchair, contact a health care specialist who can design a proper fit. You might find a wheelchair at a garage sale or receive one as a gift, but wheelchairs that do not fit properly can lead to bruises, pressure ulcers, poor posture, and other problems that can actually exacerbate your arthritis pain. Situations sometimes make it necessary to get a wheelchair immediately. If this is the case, consider borrowing or renting a chair for the short-term.

Three-wheelers, also known as scooters, are beneficial for people who can walk short spans but need help for long distances. Scooters are good for traveling over most indoor and outdoor surfaces. Most can achieve speeds up to 4 mph and have rotating seats for easy entry and exit. You can steer them with a handlebar, steering wheel, joystick, or push-button controls.

Moneysaver
Before buying or accepting any item, try it out and make sure it works properly. Sit in a wheelchair and make sure it moves smoothly and that the brakes work. Find out the store or catalog return policy. Save your receipt or cancelled check for proof of purchase and the catalog for reference.

Paying for assistive devices

Often the person who needs an assistive device is already living on a fixed income, and these devices can become a financial hardship. There are resources to help you though:

- **Your health insurance company.** See if the device is covered before buying it. Most likely, little gadgets to help around the kitchen probably are not covered, but wheelchairs, scooters and the more expensive devices may be covered either partially or totally.

- **Local health organizations.** Many get donations of used items and they recycle them back to others who may need them. Call your local hospital to get names of these organizations in your area.

Accessible housing

The need for accessible homes is growing, as is the number of older Americans who purchased their homes when they were much younger and relatively healthier and hoped to spend most of their lives there. Unexpected disabilities, such as arthritis, can force an owner to sell a home and move into one that is more accessible to meet their needs.

For example, in a two-story home, stairs can become more difficult to climb when you have arthritis. As a result, you can become confined to one-level living. Unless money is available for extensive remodeling, you are faced with the decision of selling your home and relocating to a less expensive, one-level structure. Don't pack yet—there are solutions to your problem.

"

Sometimes when all my various joints and muscles are acting up, I find that wearing high-top athletic shoes, which support my ankles, really help me to stay on my feet and be active. Velcro closures are a good solution for stiff hands too.
—Cathy, 50

Unofficially...
Medical care costs of people with rheumatoid arthritis and osteoarthritis are two to three times higher than those without arthritis, states the Mayo Clinic. People with arthritis also had more charges for procedures, hospital care, imaging studies, physician services, laboratory tests, and prescription drugs.

Modifying your current home

Whether you rent or own a home, federal law allows you to modify your current residence to accommodate your disability. In 1986, Congress passed the Fair Housing Act that protects anyone who has physical or mental impairments that substantially limit one or more major life activity, anyone who has a record of having such an impairment or are regarded by others as having such an impairment. It includes the following provisions:

- Reasonable accommodations in rules, policies, and services must be allowed so that people may more fully use and enjoy their housing.

- Individuals must be allowed to make reasonable changes to their housing at their own expense. (This does not mean structural changes, such as adding on a room, but perhaps changing round door knobs to lever door knobs.)

- It is illegal for anyone directly or indirectly involved in the sale or rental of housing or housing lots to discriminate in the sale, rental, negotiation, or inspection of housing and the terms, rates, privileges, or conditions of financing, advertising, or provisions of real estate brokerage services.

Another law that protects your rights is the American Disabilities Act (ADA), signed into law on July 26, 1990. It prohibits discrimination on the basis of disability in employment; programs and services provided by state and local governments; goods and services provided by private companies; and in commercial facilities.

It contains requirements for new construction, for alterations or renovations to buildings and facilities, and for improving access to existing facilities of private companies providing goods or services to the public. It also requires that state and local governments provide access to programs offered to the public. The ADA also covers effective communication with people with disabilities eligibility criteria that may restrict or prevent access, and requires reasonable modifications of policies and practices that may be discriminatory.

Building or buying an accessible home

If you have the finances to build a new home, you can have your needs accommodated. For example, architects can design homes with lower kitchen counters, rotating pantries, and more.

If you want to build such a home, contact a builder or architect who has experience building accessible housing and ask for references. If your state requires licensing, make sure the builder is licensed and ask for proof. You can also call your local builders association for references. Make certain that:

- You put everything you want in writing.

- Your builder has workman's compensation insurance; make sure he proves it to prevent your liability if someone gets hurt on the job.

- Your needs are met and you have a good communication with your builder.

There are now several programs that help disabled people and their families obtain financing for accessible housing. In 1996, Fannie Mae announced HomeChoice, a three-year underwriting initiative to provide single-family mortgages for low- and moderate-income borrowers with disabilities, or borrowers with a disabled family member. Check with your local Fannie Mae lender or check out the web site at http://www.fanniemae.com.

Bright Idea
If you have difficulty walking 200 feet without stopping to rest or you cannot walk without the use of a cane, wheelchair, or other assistive device, you are eligible to receive a handicapped parking sticker. For more information, contact your local motor vehicle office. You may have to supply proof of your disability. Many people misuse these stickers. Do not be one of them.

Moneysaver
New York State law grants property and school tax exemptions to homeowners with disabilities that limit one major life function, and who are receiving either Social Security Disability benefits or are legally blind. There are income limitations and this exemption is at the discretion of the individual municipalities. Check with your state to see if you qualify for any special tax breaks.

Before you build, buy, or rent another home, think about what kind of home is appropriate for you:

- **Condominiums and townhouses.** Condominiums and townhouses are multi-unit housing that provide interaction with other neighbors. The owner is required to maintain the interior of the home, but not the outside grounds. Instead, homeowners pay additional fees to the homeowners association for hired help to maintain the outside grounds (also called the common grounds). This will release the physical burden of maintaining most of the property.

- **Single-family residential homes.** It is the responsibility of the homeowner to maintain the interior and exterior of the home, and the property. Whether you own a single-family residential home, a condominium, or a townhouse, home ownership provides tax incentives and a buildup of equity. You can purchase a single-family residential unit, but you might consider budgeting additional money for a handyman to maintain the property when you are unable to do so.

- **Shared housing.** Some disabled persons have combined their resources to purchase a home together and to share similar support services. Again, each individual's situation is unique and an agreement on responsibilities and expectations should be agreed upon before moving in together.

Getting the help you need

When you were a child learning how to do something for the first time, you might have gotten frustrated and given up. Your teacher and parents taught you that when you are learning something it is okay to ask for help. As adults, we shamefully forget this and try to do it all on our own. We were taught to be independent, but even as an adult it is still okay to ask for help.

You need to choose what is important for you to do. For example, if you enjoy gardening, but find that mowing the lawn is a painful chore, hire a teenager to take over that responsibility.

If it is difficult for you to get around, a licensed care professional can bring the medical care to you. Home health care covers the use of assistive devices, such as canes, walkers, or crutches. Check with your health care plan to see if they cover in-home care.

An occupational therapist might help too. According to the American Occupational Therapist Association, occupational therapy uses everyday activities as the means of helping people to achieve independence.

For the person with a physical disability, the first focus is on performing critical daily activities, such as dressing, grooming, bathing, and eating. Once these skills are mastered, the occupational therapy program is built around the skills needed to perform a person's daily responsibilities, such as caring for a home and family, participating in school, or seeking and holding employment. Again, check with your health plan to see if using an occupational therapist is covered.

Coping on the job

For some employees, arthritis might not be affecting their jobs at all. For others, arthritis can cost them their jobs. Think about the factory worker whose gnarled fingers prevent him from tightening

Timesaver
Do not wait until you have a flare-up to find somebody to help. Ask relatives or neighbors if they would be interested in helping when your arthritis flares up. You might find a stay-at-home parent who is willing to make extra money when you need the assistance, or you might find a whole community willing to pitch in when you cannot go at it alone.

a screw on a new toy, or the waitress with osteoarthritis in her legs and feet.

Disability benefits

According to the Social Security Administration (SSA), disability under the terms defined by this organization is based on your inability to work. You will be considered disabled if you are unable to do any kind of work for which you are suited and your disability is expected to last for a least a year or can result in death.

The SSA wants to help people who want to work. Getting disability payments does not mean that you need to sit at home. The SSA has programs to help place you in a job. You can receive Social Security–disability benefits at any age, but there are special rules to determine if you are disabled. Children can also receive Social Security benefits, so children who suffer from juvenile rheumatoid arthritis might be eligible. Contact your local Social Security office for more information.

Computing in comfort

Sitting at a computer screen for long periods of time, or keeping your hands in one position can trigger flare-ups in your arthritis pain. Here are some tips to help prevent flare-ups at your desk job:

- Get up and stretch at least once an hour, including your fingers.

- Use voice-activated software that can eliminate excessive typing. You speak into a microphone, the computer recognizes your voice, and types what you are saying.

- Use an ergonomic keyboard. Although these fragmented keyboards are funny looking, the main idea behind them is to allow your hands to bend in a more natural state while typing, which prevents stiffness.

■ Use a keyboard and mouse support. These supports are pads that sit under your wrist while you type or use the computer's mouse. It props and cushions your wrist instead of having it rest on the edge of a table.

■ Make sure your computer is at the correct height. When using the computer, make sure the screen and the desk are at the correct height for your body. Your elbows should be at right angles and your shoulders should not be hunched.

Surviving stress

Stress can cause a host of physical problems, including chronic fatigue, back pain and headaches. Stress causes spasmodic pains in the neck and shoulders, musculoskeletal aches, lower back pain, and various minor muscular twitches, such as nervous tics, are more noticeable under stress.

Here are some tips to help you decrease the amount of stress in your life:

■ Identify the stressors and make lifestyle changes to eliminate them.

■ Learn quick stress-busting techniques to use at work or at home.

■ Stretch. It relieves tense muscles and improves the body's overall flexibility.

■ Stand up straight. Slouching restricts breathing and impedes circulation.

■ Uncross your legs. It reduces blood flow to the calves and feet, misaligns your pelvis, and puts pressure on your lower back. All of this pressure on your joints can contribute to flare-ups.

Bright Idea
Holding the telephone can be painful on your neck and shoulders, cause stiffness and contribute to arthritis flare-ups. Instead, invest in a telephone head set or a speakerphone to eliminate the precarious position of carrying the phone.

Unofficially...
Researchers at the Arizona State University's Department of Clinical Psychology studied the link between stress and autoimmune diseases. Fifty RA patients were monitored over two years. They had histories of increased stress and RA flare-ups. About one-third had identifiable stress episodes that led to disease activity.

- Move around every half-hour for at least a minute to prevent stiffness in the joints.

- Exercise. Regular aerobic activity reduces anxiety because it actually challenges the body's chemistry. It stimulates the brain's production of the hormone norepinephrine, which is directly related to emotional stability. Working out also activates endorphins, which are substances in the brain that provide feelings of pleasure.

- Seek professional help if stress becomes overwhelming.

- Have a massage. Scientific evidence supports the theory that touch promotes healing and relaxation, but the best part of a massage is how it feels! A wide variety of techniques are available to the consumer, the most common being standard Swedish massage and Japanese finger pressure massage, or Shiatsu. Massage not only alleviates physical and mental irritations but also promotes improved circulation, elasticity, and recovery from fatigue and muscle soreness.

- Relax. Sit down, read a book, listen to music, or rent a movie. Just relaxing at least an hour each day can eliminate much of the stress in your life. Find something that relaxes you and make time to do it on a daily basis.

- Laughter really is good medicine. Just ask Norman Cousins, who was one of the first to link the therapeutic effects of humor and laughter almost two decades ago when he described his utilization of laughter during his treatment for ankylosing spondylitis. Cousins believed that negative emotions had a negative impact on his health and that positive emotions had a positive effect. He spent the last 12 years of his life at UCLA Medical School in the Department of Behavioral Medicine exploring the scientific proof of his beliefs. He established the Humor Research Task Force, which coordinated and supported world-wide clinical research on humor.

What science has found is that laughter stimulates the immune system, which can battle the effects of stress. So watch your favorite stand-up comic, tune into an old Abbott and Costello movie, or whatever makes you laugh. It is free therapeutic medicine.

■ Delegate responsibility. If you have family members, do not do all the housework on your own. Assign chores to the kids or your spouse.

Chronic pain and fatigue are, in themselves, powerful stressors, and living with them can lead to depression. Watch for these warning signs:

■ Excessive use of drugs or alcohol.

■ Personality changes, withdrawal from social activities.

■ Ongoing feeling of sadness.

■ Thoughts of suicide.

Contact a doctor, hospital, psychologist, social worker, or mental health center immediately if you feel depressed or that you may harm yourself or others.

Arthritis and pregnancy

If you are taking any medications to help with your arthritis, it is important to know that some of these medications can cross the placenta, the protective barrier surrounding the baby, and enter into the fetus' bloodstream. Depending on the amount of drug that is passed on to the baby, the consequences can range from various birth defects to death. If you are planning to become pregnant or already are pregnant, ask your doctor whether you should refrain from using your medication. Also ask when you can resume taking the medication. If you plan on breastfeeding, ask if the medication can be passed in your milk to the baby.

Arthritis and family

When you have arthritis, your entire family may suffer. Children have to take on extra duties when you have flare-ups. If there is a child with arthritis in the family, other siblings may feel jealous or angry that they have to do a share of the child's work. They may also feel that the child with the arthritis receives more attention than they do. How can your family work together?

- Talk with your family. Explain that you may have bad days and you will try not to take it out on them. Explain what "remissions" are but do not try to make up for lost time during a "feel good" period. It might leave you feeling more pain afterward.

- Accept your bad days. Perhaps you cannot play baseball with your child as much as you would like, but you could rent a video and pop popcorn. Look for alternative things to do when you are experiencing a flare-up.

Arthritis and sexuality

If you have arthritis, you might not be very interested in sex, or are less able to have sex because of chronic pain or fatigue. Your relationship with your partner might be suffering if either or both of you are frustrated, depressed, angered, or confused about these feelings. After all, both of you understand that having arthritis is not something you wished for, but it might be preventing you from having a healthy, satisfying sexual relationship. How?

■ Low self-esteem: Swollen joints, gnarled fingers or a noticeable change in your walk can make you feel unattractive and cause your self-esteem to suffer. In addition, the inability to feel independent at times may also affect your self-esteem.

■ Fatigue: You are just too pooped to make love.

■ Pain: Medications can decrease lubrication in the vagina causing intercourse to be uncomfortable. Even if penetration is not painful, different positions may put pressure on your joints.

■ Medical problems: Some forms of arthritis can trigger additional medical complications. For example, lupus can cause oral or vaginal ulcers, and medications can also inhibit your sexual drive. This is common with Sjogren's syndrome, as well. A vaginal lubricant can help to make intercourse easier.

How can you create a better relationship between you and your partner?

■ Work on feeling good. Feeling good takes work, so choose flattering clothes and a haircut that is easy to care for. Discover what makes you feel good and make that part of your daily routine, whether it is a special fragrance or a sexy nightgown.

Bright Idea
There are never enough tips for living easier with arthritis. For 250 more, contact the New York Arthritis Exchange, Pfizer Inc.: 212-984-8730; or from the 914 code only: 800-246-2884.

- Talk it out. Communication between partners is vital for a healthy relationship, especially a sexual relationship. Talk to your partner and tell him that you need reassurance and support when having sex is difficult for you. Make sure both of you understand that there is more to making love than intercourse, but sometimes cuddling might be it for that night.

- Plan for sex. Many times sex takes place at night, but if you experience chronic pain and fatigue during the day, sex is not on your mind by nightfall. Instead, get out your appointment book and plan for a midday rendezvous or an early weekend morning when you and your partner can concentrate on nothing but being together. Do not, however, feel forced to have intercourse during this time. Concentrate on what feels good and what you can do, not what you cannot do.

- Take pain medication and a warm bath beforehand to help loosen your joints, and make you feel more comfortable.

- Understand your partner's feelings. When you marry, you might have declared your love "in sickness and in health" and at times that dedication is put to the test. Your partner might want to help you but does not know how. He may not be sure when to step in and help without hurting your independence or self-confidence. Let him know what he can do for you.

Using your joints wisely

If you hurt your back, you would not pick up a box, right? Using your back muscles wisely would prevent further pain and injury. This is the same idea when you have arthritis. It is important to know how to use your joints properly so they are not coping with additional stress and strain.

- Lose weight. Removing additional weight from your arthritic joints reduces joint irritation.

- Watch your hands and other muscles. When you are stressed, you probably clench your fists. Becoming conscious of these activities will also limit any undue stress. Also avoid tight or twisting motions. For example, instead of using your entire hand to open a jar, lean on a screw top jar with the palm of your hand and turn the lid with a shoulder motion to reduce stress to your fingers.

- Plan. Think about what you need to do in one day and plan it out. Give yourself plenty of breaks and alternate heavier tasks with light tasks. For example, do not attempt to go grocery shopping and wash your car all in the same day. It might be to much on your joints.

- Organize. Combine steps and find shortcuts to doing things. For example, choose one day to prepare a few days' meals that can be frozen, so on days you are not up to cooking, you still have a nutritious meal to look forward to.

- Think it out. If an activity is causing pain, stop doing it: It is that simple. Think about what you are doing before you do it. Think about keeping a straight posture and concentrate on loosening tight muscles. If you know that one position is going to aggravate your arthritis, remind yourself to move around.

If you already experiencing a flare-up, try to pinpoint what activity might have contributed to the pain.

66

I do have to cater my schedule around my condition. I guess I've been doing it for so long, I just do it. People who don't have arthritis or pain can't seem to understand what it's like. You look okay, but they wonder why are you so slow or tired, or poop out fast.
—Joan, 48.

99

- Accept the pain. Once you accept the fact that you are experiencing a flare-up or chronic pain, you may try to find methods that help you to cope. For example, on days that you cannot go shopping at the mall, can you scan the catalogs that have been piling up at home? Can you shop on the Internet instead, or watch any of the cable shopping networks? If grocery shopping is out of the question, how about pizza delivery? Taking off a night to pamper yourself when you are not feeling well can do a world of good in your recuperation.

Just the facts

- The pain and chronic fatigue of arthritis can interfere with your day-to-day living, but there are steps you can take to keep it from moving you to the sidelines of life.

- Assistive devices like wheelchairs, scooters, and walkers are frequently covered by insurance.

- The Fair Housing Act and the Americans with Disabilities Act protects your rights to accessible housing, and to modify your existing home to accommodate your arthritis-related disabilities.

- Stress exacerbates arthritic aches and pains—it's important to reduce stress in your lifestyle wherever possible.

- Regular exercise is key to reducing your susceptibility to arthritis pain. Maintain a regular regimen of low-impact exercise.

Support Groups and Treatment

W hen Janet was diagnosed with fibromyalgia, she felt alone and scared. She had many questions about having fibromyalgia, but did not know anyone she could talk to who shared her condition. She searched for a local fibromyalgia support group, but the nearest one was too far away for her to attend regularly. Finally, Janet contacted her local branch of the Arthritis Foundation, and they helped Janet to organize a support group closer to her area.

Janet remembers the first fibromyalgia support group meeting well. "The room was filled with about 60 people of all ages," says the 63-year-old. "Then a teenager, way in the back of the room, stood up and simply asked, 'When am I going to feel better?' Everyone in the room knew exactly how this 17-year-old felt."

"Since that first meeting, we have developed a bond with each other," says Janet. "These meetings are something we look forward to. We always have

Chapter 15

the opportunity to raise issues that might be personal, such as reactions to medication that we may be having, any physical complaints, and the oh, so many little things that occur with fibromyalgia."

Now the support group meets monthly, discusses their conditions, and tackles new coping mechanisms, such as guided imagery, yoga exercise, stress management, dance therapy, and t'ai chi. "It is a very positive feeling when people come in smiling and greeting each other," says Janet. "It is not always the exact same group from month to month, but there is a familiarity with each other."

You are not alone

A support group like Janet's is a group of people with a common condition meeting on a regular basis to share stories, advice, and emotional support. Support groups can also be a forum to learn practical information about your condition, such as the most recent medical information, or the latest diagnostic technology.

Depending on your circumstances and personality, it may be beneficial to turn to others for help. You may feel less alone with your illness when talking with others who face or have faced similar challenges.

If a face-to-face support group is not for you, you may want to try one of the many online support groups. Here you can chat with people who have the same condition as you, but in the privacy and comfort of your own home.

This chapter will discuss finding a support group that works for you. You may even discover that you need professional support, so it is also important to know how to find a professional counselor or psychologist. Whatever you choose to use, it is most important that you are comfortable in your decision.

How support groups work

In general, support groups are moderated by either:

- a medical professional, such as a nurse, social worker, physician, or psychologist; or,

- group members, who are often called peer or self-help groups.

Some groups are designed to be more educational and structured. They may invite a physician to lecture on a new treatment or study. Some groups emphasize emotional support and shared experiences, but do not discuss medical treatments. Some concentrate only on a specific type of arthritis (rheumatoid, osteoarthritis, or lupus, for instance) while others are more inclusive.

Cyberlife support groups

In addition to traditional face-to-face support groups, the Internet offers online "virtual" support groups and communities.

Tina is 33 and has rheumatoid arthritis. When she was first diagnosed, she checked for local support groups, but they were held at senior centers or retirement communities. "I have nothing against seniors, but feel that the problems I faced at that time, as a working mother, are much different than an 80-year-old retired person! So I didn't attend any of the groups."

Instead she started http://www.ArthritisNet.com for anyone who has arthritis or those with a loved one who has it. "I try to put the information in layman's terms. I am a nurse and when I started researching arthritis on the web, I couldn't understand the 'doctorese' language used at many of the

Unofficially...
According to Dr. Ronald C. Kessler at Harvard, self-help groups have become one of the most important de facto treatments for dealing with emotional problems in the U.S. Their popularity has outstripped more conventional sources of help, including psychiatrists, psychologists, and even ministers. Nearly 19 percent of all participants in his study reported seeking help through such a venue.

web sites. If I couldn't understand then probably many other people didn't either!"

ArthritisNet.com is one of many arthritis web pages and is still under construction, but offers brief descriptions of many forms of arthritis, information on medication, bulletin boards to exchange information, news on medications or alternative treatments, areas to find a pen pal or mentor, links to other web sites with more information, tips to make household tasks easier, a chat room for scheduled chats for adults and kids with arthritis, and a special kids section. Tina also e-mails a newsletter on a regular basis.

Tina admits that if you are looking for scientific information, you should look elsewhere. She calls ArthritisNet.com for the "average Joe." "I had two complaints that the newsletter is too "chatty." I told those people to look elsewhere. Chattiness, friendliness, support, is what it's all about!" she says.

"I was going to have a synovectomy on eight joints of my right hand," says Tina. "Well, how many people do you know that have had a synovectomy? I knew *none* in "real" life. But in "cyber" life, I knew plenty! They told me what to expect and what recovery would be like. They knew; they had been there. And my e-mail box was filled with get well wishes. Just knowing *that* many people care, well you have to heal faster with so many good thoughts!"

Online support groups also include:

- **Newsgroups:** a "virtual" bulletin board, with lists of messages on similar topics posted by users. You can read some or all the messages (called posts). You can post a message or simply "browse" the list.

- **Listservers:** different from newsgroups and operated by private e-mail. You actually "join" a listserv, and, as a member, you receive e-mails on a similar topic from other members. Each time anyone in the group sends an e-mail, you get a copy. If you send an e-mail, a copy goes to everyone.

But be careful. You do not know who else is online with you. Online support groups are an excellent source of practical advice or emotional support, but can also be a source of incorrect or possibly harmful medical information. Look for groups affiliated with a reputable organization or hosted by an expert. If you have any questions about treatments or advice discussed, ask your doctor.

There are also dozens of documented instances of people who have faked their way into Internet support groups. Unfortunately, the victims of fakers in Internet support groups end up growing suspicious of one another and are often hurt, angry, and embarrassed. If you become suspicious of someone's story on the Internet, contact the monitor of that forum or web page and alert them immediately.

If you are not computer savvy, consider other forms of emotional support:

- Round-robin groups: where you write personal letters to each other.

- Telephone-conference support groups.

- One-on-one counseling.

You do not have to depend on just one form of support either. Perhaps you enjoy talking with a group of people, but prefer to have some privacy on other issues. You may combine support groups and one-on-one counseling.

For more information on online support groups: contact The American Self-Help Clearinghouse: St. Claire's Hospital, Denville, N.J.

> **"**
> I began the PsoriaticArthritis ONELIST Mailing group to give us PA'ers a forum just for us. It is an e-mail only list, so there is no direct chatting, unless people choose to do so privately. Currently, after only two months, we have 45-plus members from all over the world! We discuss personal histories, treatments, current situations, symptoms, and any other PA related topic that interests us.
> —Michelle, 38
> **"**

07834-2995. It offers help in locating and forming self-help groups. Two other online resources to check out are Support-Group.com and http://www.dejanews.com

Finding a support group

Support groups are not necessarily listed in the Yellow Pages. To find a support group:

- Ask a health care provider for assistance. A doctor, nurse, social worker, chaplain, or psychologist may be able to refer you to one.
- You can check the telephone book or newspaper for a listing of support resources.
- Contact community centers, libraries, churches, or synagogues in your area. This is where many support group meetings are held or information is posted.
- Ask others you know with arthritis for suggestions.
- Contact a state or national arthritis organization, such as The Arthritis Foundation.
- Search the Internet. Many state and national arthritis organizations have web sites that offer information on local support groups. Most support groups are free, collect voluntary donations, or charge only modest membership dues to cover expenses.

Choosing a support group

Choosing a support group that is right for you depends on several factors, but the key is finding a group that matches your needs and personality.

If you decide to take part in a group (real or virtual), try it out a few times. You may have to experiment with different kinds of support groups before you find one that meets your needs. If you do not find it useful or comfortable, do not feel obligated to continue or to speak. You may gain just from listening. Avoid any groups that promise a cure or suggest that support groups are a substitute for medical treatment.

Starting a support group

Tess, a 52-year-old woman with lupus, developed a support group for similarly afflicted people in her area. "I was diagnosed with lupus in 1983, but the problem wasn't just having the lupus, but with other people's attitudes about the condition," she says. "Many thought that if I just think positively I would get better. They didn't understand. It was important to me to talk to other people and help them through these attitudes."

"Sometimes we have people spilling their guts about their feelings and other times we talk about the things going on in our family. Sometimes we have a doctor come in to talk about lupus."

Here are some tips for starting your own support group, whether virtual or real:

- Before starting from scratch, see if a group already exists. Contact a national group and ask for any local affiliates or a packet on how to get started. Do an Internet search to see what other online groups already exist.

- Get ideas by attending a meeting of other support groups that may be somewhat similar to your group.

- Find a suitable meeting place and time. There is usually free space at a local church, library, community center, hospital, or social service agency. If the group is small enough, you may

> 66
> If you don't feel comfortable, you shouldn't have to go back. The people here have a lot of issues, but the rule is that whatever is being said is no one else's business. It stays in the four walls,
> —Tess, 52.
> 99

want to have the meeting at members homes and rotate the home each time you meet.

If you are starting an online group, determine if a live chat would be more successful than a message board. Start a message thread to see what the needs are.

Publicize and run the first meeting. Send notices to the newspapers, radio, magazines, and television stations in your area about your meeting at least three weeks in advance. Many of these venues will provide free advertising to not-for-profit groups.

If you are organizing an online conference, publicize the conference through the systems operator or by sending e-mail messages to those who have expressed interest in your group. Follow through after the meeting and ask for feedback. Here are some additional tips:

- Use professionals. Find an expert on your topic in your area and ask if they could speak to your group and answer any questions they may have.

- Stay in touch with members. Find a way to stay in touch with your members between meetings, whether it is a phone list, newsletter or e-mail system.

- Do not have overly high expectations. Expect your group to experience ups and downs in terms of attendance and enthusiasm. It will also depend on weather and time of year. For example, do not plan your first meeting around a holiday and expect bad weather to decrease attendance.

- Be patient. Whether you are organizing a real-life or virtual support group, you need to be patient and supportive of the people who are attending your meetings or reading your postings. Remember, they are there for support.

Not for everyone

Support groups are not for everyone. When you have arthritis, a strong friend and family network is important and may be enough for you. One recent study of breast cancer support groups by researchers at Carnegie-Mellon University found that attending a support group actually did more harm than good for women with breast cancer who had close social ties (family, friends, their faith). Some of these women found it depressing to talk to women who were sicker than they were. However, that study also found that women who were not getting enough emotional support from their families, friends, and doctors *did* benefit from support groups, so it is important to determine exactly what your emotional needs are. Support groups can be highly beneficial and may be worth exploring during any stage of your illness or treatment.

Consider therapy

At some time in our lives, each of us may feel overwhelmed and may need help dealing with our problems. After all, having arthritis can be debilitating and can take over your life. You may be so tired of taking medications, going to doctor's appointments, and trying new treatments that are not helping your pain.

According to psychologist and researcher Gail Wright of the Truman Memorial Veterans Hospital in Columbia, Missouri, it is estimated that one in four people with rheumatoid arthritis has some form of depression. Wright researched the relationship between arthritis and depression at Truman

I have lupus, but I do not go to any support groups. I have a wonderful husband, and am very connected with my church, so I get support there. I don't define myself by lupus and getting involved with lupus activities would, to me, be letting the disease win mentally...it's not who I am by a long shot.
—Joanne, 45

Memorial Veterans Hospital, and found that between 14 and 27 percent of adults with rheumatoid arthritis are depressed, while only 5 percent of the general population exhibits the same signs. Individuals with the painful musculoskeletal condition fibromyalgia have higher rates of depression, though children with juvenile arthritis exhibit about the same rate of depression as others their age.

Perhaps you just cannot handle your illness anymore or your family is having a difficult time adjusting. According to the National Institute of Mental Health (NIMH), more than 30 million Americans need help dealing with feelings and problems that seem beyond their control— problems with a marriage or relationship, a family situation, or dealing with losing a job, the death of a loved one, depression, stress, burnout, or substance abuse. Those losses and stresses of daily living can at times be significantly debilitating.

At times we need outside help from a trained, licensed professional in order to work through these problems. Through therapy, psychologists help millions of Americans of all ages live healthier, more productive lives.
The NIMH suggests that you consider professional therapy if:

- You feel an overwhelming and prolonged sense of helplessness and sadness, and your problems do not seem to get better despite your efforts and help from family and friends.

- You are finding it difficult to carry out everyday activities. For example, you are unable to concentrate on assignments at work, and your job performance is suffering as a result.

- You worry excessively, expect the worst, or are constantly on edge.

- Your actions are harmful to yourself or to others. For instance, you are drinking too much alcohol, abusing drugs, or becoming overly argumentative and aggressive.

Counselors

According to the American Counseling Association, professional counselors undergo extensive education and training, which includes at least a master's degree and field training with a solid foundation in human growth and development, career and lifestyle development, social and cultural foundations, and group work, private practice, and internships. Forty-four states and the District of Columbia require counselors to hold a license. Professional counselors serve at all levels of schools and universities, in hospitals, mental health agencies, rehabilitation facilities, business and industry, correctional institutions, religious organizations, community centers, and private practice.

Common ways to locate a counselor include:

- Referral from physician.

- National Board for Certified Counselors referral service (336) 547-0607.

  Established in 1981, NBCC has certified over 18,000 counselors in the general practice of counseling. This general practice credential is appropriate for all counselors who have earned a minimum of a master's degree and have demonstrated minimum competence levels considered to be important for all counselors. It is assumed that all counselors, regardless of their specialty area(s), must have a shared knowledge base and be able to perform some of the same activities.

- Friends or family members.
- Crisis hot lines.
- Community mental health agencies.
- Local United Way information and referral service.
- Hospitals.
- Government social services.
- Schools, colleges, and universities.
- Clergy.

Psychologists and psychotherapy

Psychotherapy helps you talk openly and confidentially about your concerns and feelings. Psychologists who specialize in psychotherapy and other forms of psychological treatment are highly trained professionals with expertise in the areas of human behavior, mental health assessment, diagnosis and treatment, and behavioral changes. Psychologists work with patients to alter their feelings and attitudes and help them develop healthier, more effective patterns of behavior.

Psychologists apply scientifically validated procedures to help people change their thoughts, emotions, and behaviors. Studies show that some forms of psychotherapy can effectively decrease depression, anxiety, and related symptoms, such as pain, fatigue, and nausea.

There is also evidence that most people who have at least several sessions of psychotherapy are far better off than individuals with emotional difficulties who are untreated.

Finding a psychologist

The American Psychological Association (APA) located in Washington, D.C., is the largest scientific and professional organization representing psychology in the United States and is the world's largest association of psychologists. APA's membership includes more than 132,000 practitioners, researchers, educators, consultants, and students. Through its divisions in 49 subfields of psychology and affiliations with 57 state and Canadian provincial associations, APA works to advance psychology as a science, as a profession, and as a means of promoting human welfare. For more information on psychologists or psychology, contact the APA at American Psychological Association, Office of Public Affairs, Washington, DC 20002-4242, (202) 336-5700 or e-mail: public.affairs@apa.org.

To find a psychologist, you can also ask your physician or another health professional, consult a local university or college department of psychology, ask family and friends, or contact your area community mental health center.

Questions to ask

The APA suggests asking a psychologist the following questions before beginning counseling with him or her: "Are you a licensed psychologist?" and "How many years have you been practicing psychology?"

The American Psychological Association states that after graduation from college, psychologists spend an average of seven years in graduate education training and research before receiving a doctoral degree. As part of their professional training, they must complete a supervised clinical internship in a hospital or organized health setting and at least one year of post-doctoral supervised experience before they can practice independently in any health care arena.

By law, psychologists must be licensed by the state or jurisdiction in which they practice. In most states, renewal of this license depends upon the demonstration of continued competence and requires continuing education. In addition, members of the APA adhere to a strict code of professional ethics.

Additional questions to ask would include:

▪ I have been feeling (anxious, tense, depressed, etc.), and I'm having problems (with my job, my marriage, eating, sleeping, etc.). What experience do you have helping people with these types of problems?

▪ What are your areas of expertise? (For example, working with children and families.)

▪ What kinds of treatments do you use, and have they been proven effective for dealing with my kind of problem or issue?

▪ What are your fees? (Fees are usually based on a 45-minute to 50-minute session.) Do you have a sliding-scale fee policy? How much therapy would you recommend?

▪ What types of insurance do you accept? Will you accept direct billing to/payment from my insurance company? Are you affiliated with any managed care organizations? Do you accept Medicare/Medicaid insurance?

Finally, the most important factor in determining whether to work with a particular psychologist—once that psychologist's credentials and competence have been established—is your level of personal comfort with that psychologist. A good rapport with your psychologist is critical. Choose a psychologist with whom you feel comfortable and at ease.

Paying for it

Many insurance companies provide coverage for mental health services. If you have private health insurance coverage (typically through an employer), check with your insurance company to see if mental health services are covered and, if so, how you may obtain these benefits. Find out how much the insurance company will reimburse for mental health services and what limitations on the use of benefits may apply.

If you are not covered, you may decide to pay for psychological services out-of-pocket. Some psychologists operate on a sliding-scale fee policy, where the amount you pay depends on your income.

Another potential source of mental health services involves government-sponsored health care programs, including Medicare for individuals aged 65 or older, as well as health insurance plans for government employees, military personnel, and their dependents. Community mental health centers throughout the country are another possible alternative for receiving mental health services. And, some state Medicaid programs for economically disadvantaged individuals provide for limited mental health services from psychologists.

How will I know if the therapy is working?

As you begin, you should have clear goals established with your psychologist. You might be trying to overcome feelings of hopelessness associated with

Moneysaver
Local support groups are usually free of charge. Check out the support groups in your area to help save money instead of using costly medical professionals. Of course, if you are depressed or feel that you are a danger to yourself or someone else, do not sacrifice money for safety. Contact a professional immediately.

depression. Remember, certain goals require more time to reach than others. You and your psychologist should decide at what point you may expect to begin to see progress.

People often feel a wide variety of emotions during psychotherapy. Some people have qualms about therapy that result from their difficulty discussing painful and troubling experiences. When you begin to feel relief or hope, it can actually be a positive sign indicating that you are starting to explore your thoughts and behavior.

Resources

Contact the American Self-Help Clearinghouse, a department of the Behavioral Health Center of Saint Clare's Health Services in Denville, NJ, for a 344-page Self-Help Sourcebook, available for $7.20 (a 40 percent Internet discount, add $4 for overseas airmail) by sending a check to: American Self-Help Clearinghouse, Attn.: SB, St. Clare's Hospital, Denville, NJ 07834-2995.

There are descriptions for groups that contain either an e-mail and/or web site address. In addition to chapters on starting and understanding self-help groups, new chapters include a literature review of empirical research on groups by Dr. Keith Humphreys & Elaina Kyrouz at Stanford University; and a chapter on starting e-mail discussion groups and newsgroups by Dr. John Grohol. The introduction is by Dr. Phyllis Silverman, Department of Psychiatry, Harvard Medical School; and the Foreword by Dr. Alfred H. Katz, retired Professor Emeritus, UCLA School of Public Health.

You can reach the American Clearinghouse by phone weekdays at (973) 625-3037; TTY 625-9053 for hearing impaired. They also run the New Jersey

Self-Help Clearinghouse, available in NJ at (800) FOR-M.A.S.H. (Mutual Aid Self-Help) or (800) 367-6274.

Just the facts

- Not everyone needs a support group, but if you feel better talking with someone who shares the same condition, it might be beneficial.

- Be patient. Talking with someone does not change things in one meeting. It may take meeting regularly to feel better.

- If you feel that your life or your feelings are out of control, contact a mental health professional.

- Do not give anyone personal information about yourself, including addresses, credit card numbers, or phone numbers, when you are online.

Glossary

Acupressure A Chinese medical treatment that uses hands-on pressure to certain points on the body that alleviates ailments or pain.

Acupuncture The ancient practice of inserting very fine needles into the skin to stimulate certain points in the body. Heat (moxibustion), pressure, friction, suction (cupping), or electromagnetic energy (electro-acupuncture) are used on the needles as well.

Allopurinol A drug used to prevent gout attacks and kidney stones caused by uric acid.

Ankylosing spondylitis A disease that joins the bones of the spinal column together. There is a strong chance that it can be inherited. The hips, shoulders, neck, ribs, and jaw can be affected as well. Treatment includes pain relief, physical therapy, and possibly surgery.

Antibiotic Medications that have the ability to kill or prevent the growth of a living organism. They are used to treat infections.

Antimalarial drug A drug that kills or prevents the growth of malaria, but is now used as a treatment to reduce pain symptoms of arthritis.

313

Aromatherapy Alternative therapy that uses chemical scents from natural herbs, extracts, and oils to relieve symptoms and boost the immune system.

Arthritis A general term used to describe more than 100 different rheumatic diseases that affect the joints, muscles, and connective tissues of the body. The two most prevalent forms of arthritis are osteoarthritis (OA) and rheumatoid arthritis (RA).

Arthrocentesis A procedure where a joint is punctured with a needle and synovial fluid from the joint is withdrawn. Arthrocentesis is done to get samples of synovial fluid to diagnose an infection of the joint.

Arthrodesis "Freezing" of a joint through surgery, due to destruction of cartilage and bone.

Arthroscopy A surgical procedure that examines the interior of a joint with a camera-like instrument through small incisions made at the joint. The results are used to diagnose or treat joint abnormalities including torn cartilage, reconstructing ligaments, and removing inflamed joint tissues, also known as a synovectomy.

Aspirin A nonsteroidal anti-inflammatory medication that relieves pain, reduces fever, and reduces swelling and inflammation. It can also cause stomach and intestinal problems, such as ulcers and bleeding.

Beta-carotene Found in apricots, carrots, pumpkins, and spinach. Converts to vitamin A, which promotes the growth of cells and tissues in your body. A significant deficiency of vitamin A, in turn, may lead to poor growth. Too much vitamin A, however, can actually lead to reduced bone density and increase your risk of osteoporosis.

Biopsy A procedure where a small piece of living tissue is removed from a specific area of the body and examined under a microscope. Different kinds of biopsies include aspiration biopsy and needle biopsy.

Calcinosis A condition that causes deposits of calcium in the skin and muscles.

Calcium A mineral found mainly in the bones and teeth. The body needs calcium to carry nerve signals, to contract muscles, to clot blood, to help heart functions, and to work with enzymes.

Cancellous bone The spongy, inner part of many bones, mainly bones that have marrow.

Capsaicin Capsicum/cayenne peppers contain capsaicin, an irritant that produces a feeling of warmth throughout the body. Capsaicin is now a salve that has been approved by the FDA for pain relief. It does not cure arthritis, but can help to relieve its pain.

Chamomile An herb that is commonly used as a sedative, anti-spasmodic, and anti-inflammatory. Considered safe by the Food and Drug Administration, with no known side effects when used during pregnancy, during lactation, or in childhood. It is commonly used as a tea or applied as a compress.

Chiropractor A system of therapy based on the theory that a person's health depends on the condition of the musculoskeletal and nervous systems. Chiropractors usually manipulate the spinal column.

Chondrocytes Cartilage cells in the body.

Chondroitin Resembling cartilage.

Contractures An abnormal condition where a joint is bent and will not move, caused by shortening and wasting away of muscle fibers or by loss of the normal stretchiness of the skin.

Corticosteroids A hormone made in the outer layer of the adrenal gland that works with the heart and lung systems and functions of the muscles, kidneys, and other organs. These drugs are commonly referred to as steroids.

Creatinine A substance formed from the making of creatine and common in blood, urine, and muscle tissue.

Cytokines A generic term for a large group of proteins that act as chemical messengers. They enhance cell growth.

DMARDs Known as disease-modifying anti-rheumatic drugs, these drugs work to slow or stop the basic progress of the disease. They need to be taken for several weeks or months before improvement can be seen. The side effects can be great, so these medications are reserved for severe and progressive diseases.

Echinacea Also known as purple cornflower and black-eyed Susan, an herbal immune system booster and an antibiotic, which increase the chances of fighting off illnesses. It stimulates production of T-cells and enhances white blood cell function.

Endoscopy Examination of the inside of organs and cavities of the body with an endoscope.

Estrogen A group of female sex hormones. Lack of estrogen can lead to brittle bones (osteoporosis). The loss of bone density can accelerate at menopause, when your body ceases producing estrogen, a hormone needed for bone strength.

Feverfew An herb used to prevent migraines, but is now being studied as a possible treatment to reduce the symptoms of rheumatoid arthritis. Side effects of this herb include oral ulcers, headaches, allergic reaction, and gastrointestinal irritation.

Fibroblasts A cell that serves as the base for the connective or supporting tissues of the body.

Fibrositis Swelling of connective tissue; symptoms include pain and stiffness.

Fibromyalgia A syndrome of the bones, muscles, joints, and connective tissue that mimics many symptoms of arthritis. There is still a great deal to learn about this syndrome, but 18 tender points on the body have been uncovered that are common in people who have fibromyalgia.

Glucosamine A substance that is synthesized by the body and can play a role in repairing cartilage. It is believed that it may stimulate cartilage cells to grow and may inhibit the enzymes that break down this process.

Gout A disease that increases production of uric acid. Excess uric acid is converted to sodium urate crystals that settle into joints and other tissues. Symptoms include painful swelling of a joint, chills, and fever. The disease can be disabling and, if left untreated, can lead to breakdown of the joint. Treatment includes a diet that excludes purine-rich foods and pain relief medication.

Hematocrit (HCT) The measure of the number of red cells found in the blood. If your red blood cell count is low, you might be experiencing chronic inflammation, which results in pain, redness, swelling, and warmth of your joints.

Hemoglobin (Hgb) A compound in the blood that carries red blood cells and transports oxygen.

Herb A plant or part of a plant that has medicinal, aromatic, or savory qualities. Although herbs might seem "natural" or lacking in chemicals, herb plants actually produce and contain a variety of chemical substances.

Hydrotherapy Water exercises. Your body's buoyancy eliminates impact or pressure on your bones and joints, so an arthritis sufferer can move in water without pain. The water also reduces the amount of stiffness in the joint. Hydrotherapy provides good strength-training benefits.

Immunosuppressive Description of a substance or procedure that represses or prevents the immune system from responding.

Inflammation When the tissues of your body are injured or irritated, they may be inflamed. Signs include redness, heat, swelling, and pain, accompanied by loss of function.

Lyme disease An inflammatory disease, involving one or more joints, believed to be transmitted by a tick. The condition was originally discovered in Lyme, Connecticut.

Magnetic resonance imaging Medical imaging that uses radio frequency radiation to see soft tissue. It has become an important tool in the imaging of muscles and bones. Patients must remain motionless.

Meadowsweet An herbal treatment used as an antirheumatic and anti-inflammatory. May also be used to treat gout.

Menopause The period ending the female reproductive phase of life, between 45 and 60 years of age. It may stop earlier in life as a result of illness or the surgical removal of the uterus or both ovaries.

Methotrexate This is probably the most commonly prescribed DMARD for arthritis. Methotrexate is used to treat psoriasis, psoriatic arthritis, and rheumatoid arthritis.

Minocycline An antibiotic from the tetracycline family that was originally used to treat acne. When treating arthritis, minocycline is believed to block metalloproteinases, enzymes that destroy cartilage inside joints. Minocycline is also believed to suppress the immune system. Rheumatologists are uncertain as to how the antibiotic works, and more studies are needed.

Multifactorial Some forms of arthritis are multifactorial, which means that there is more than one reason for the condition.

Musculoskeletal system   The body system that includes your muscles and bones. The adult human skeletal system consists of 206 bones.

NSAIDs Known as nonsteroidal anti-inflammatory drugs, these medications slow down the body's production of prostaglandins, substances that play a role in inflammation. NSAIDs also carry some analgesic, or painkilling, properties as well. NSAIDs can cause gastrointestinal irritation.

Omega-3 acids A polyunsaturated fat found in fish that may have an anti-inflammatory effect. Omega-3 fatty acids decrease the production of the tumor necrosis factor (TNF), a protein produced in high levels in patients suffering from a chronic illness, such as rheumatoid arthritis. Can be found in seafood, especially higher-fat fish, such as albacore tuna, mackerel, and salmon, or it can be taken as a dietary supplement.

Osteoarthritis A degenerative disease of the joints of the body that affects 16 million people in the United States. Cartilage breaks down and exposes bone to rub against bone.

Osteomyelitis An infection of bone and bone marrow caused by germs that enter the bone by injury, infection, or surgery.

Osteopathy   The practice of medicine that uses drugs, surgery, and radiation, but looks more at the links between the organs and the muscle and skeletal system.

Osteotomy The surgical procedure that saws or cuts a bone. This is especially recommended treatment for ankylosing spondylitis, when there is a badly bent spine. The surgeon removes damaged bone and tissue and restores the joint to its proper position. Recovery is lengthy and osteotomy does not guarantee that the function of the joint will improve. Additional treatment may be necessary.

Periosteum A covering of the bones with an outer layer of connective tissue. Periosteum has the nerves and blood vessels that supply the bones. It is thick and rich in blood vessels over young bones but thinner and with fewer blood vessels in later life. Bones that lose periosteum through injury or disease often waste or die.

Physiatrist A physician who works in physical medicine.

Phytochemicals Substances that plants naturally produce to protect themselves against viruses, bacteria, and fungi. Different plant foods supply different kinds and amounts of phytochemicals. These foods are in vegetables, legumes, fruits, and whole grains.

Pleuritis Swelling of the linings of the lungs. Symptoms include breathlessness and stabbing pain.

Polymyositis Inflammation of muscles.

Postmenopausal Referring to the period of life following menopause.

Premenopausal Referring to the time of life before menopause.

Prostaglandin A strong hormonelike fatty acid that acts in small amounts on certain organs.

Purines The end products of digestion of proteins in the diet. Some purines are made in the body.

Purines are in many drugs and other substances, including caffeine. Too much blood uric acid may occur in people who are not able to use up and release purines, leading to gout.

Psoriasis A genetic skin disorder with red patches of thick, dry, silvery scales anywhere on the body. Psoriatic arthritis may either precede or follow this condition.

Range-of-motion Stretching exercises that help to maintain normal joint movement, and maintain or increase flexibility. These are gentle stretching exercises that help to move each joint as far as possible in all directions. They need to be done daily to help keep joints fully mobile and prevent stiffness and deformities.

Rheumatoid arthritis The immune system, in effect, turns on itself and attacks healthy joint tissue. This assault on the immune system causes inflammation of the synovium—a membrane that lines the joints. The affected cells respond to this inflammation by releasing an enzyme that can destroy the surrounding bone and cartilage. Left untreated, the joints can lose shape, resulting in pain, loss of movement, and possibly destruction of the joint.

Scleroderma A rare disease that affects the blood vessels and connective tissue. It is marked by the skin of the face and hands becoming hard.

Sed rate test Also called the erythrocyte sedimentation rate (ESR) test, it monitors how fast red blood cells cling together, fall, and settle to the bottom of a glass tube. The higher the sed rate, the greater the amount of inflammation. It helps to diagnose rheumatoid arthritis, lupus, scleroderma, systemic lupus erythematosus, Grave's disease, and other inflammatory diseases.

Serotonin Also called 5-hydroxytryptamine. A substance found naturally in the brain and intestines.

St. John's Wort An herbal remedy used to combat depression.

Support group A group of people with a common condition meeting on a regular basis to share stories, advice, and emotional support. Also a forum to learn practical information about your condition, such as the most recent medical information, or the latest diagnostic technology.

Synovectomy A surgical procedure that cuts out the synovial membrane of a joint.

Synovial fluid A clear, sticky fluid released by synovial membranes and acting as a lubricant for many joints.

Vasculitis A swelling condition of the blood vessels that is the mark of certain systemic diseases or is caused by an allergic reaction.

Resources

American Academy of Medical Acupuncture
5820 Wilshire Blvd., Suite 500
Los Angeles, CA 90036
Phone: 213-937-5514 (in California)
Toll free: 800-521-AAMA (outside California)
Web site: www.medicalacupuncture.org

American Academy of Orthopaedic Surgeons
6300 North River Road
Rosemont, IL 60018-4262
Phone: 847-823-7186
Toll free: 800-346-AAOS
Fax: 847-823-8125
Web site: Www.aaos.org

American Academy of Pain Management
13947 Mono Way, Unit A
Sonora, CA 95370
Phone: 209-533-9744

American Academy of Pediatrics
141 Northwest Point Blvd.
Elk Grove Village, IL 60007-1098
Phone: 847-228-5005
Fax: 847-228-5097
Web site: www.aap.org
E-mail: kidsdocs@aap.org

American Chronic Pain Association
P.O. Box 850
Rocklin, CA 95677
Phone: 916-632-0922
Fax: 916-632-3208
Web site: www.theacpa.org
E-mail: acpa@pacbell.net

American Chiropractic Association (ACA)
1701 Claredon Blvd.
Arlington, VA 22209
Phone: 703-276-8800
Toll free: 800-986-4636
Web site: www.amerchiro.org

American College of Rheumatology
1800 Century Place, Suite 200
Atlanta, GA 30345
Phone: 404-633-3777
Fax: 404-633-1870
Web site: www.rheumatology.org
E-mail: acr@rheumatology.org

American Pain Society
4700 West Lake Avenue
Glenview, IL 60025
Phone: 847-375-4715
Fax: 847-375-4777
Web site: www.ampainsoc.org
E-mail: info@ampainsoc.org

Arthritis Foundation
1330 West Peachtree Street
Atlanta, GA 30309
Phone: 404-872-7100 or call your local chapter
Toll free: 800-283-7800
Fax: 404-872-8694
Web site: www.arthritis.org
E-mail: help@arthritis.org

Crohn's and Colitis Foundation of America (CCFA)
386 Park Avenue South
New York, NY 10016
Phone: 212-685-3440 (in NYC)
Toll free: 800-932-2423 (outside NYC)
Fax: 212-779-4098
Web site: www.ccfa.org
E-mail: info@ccfa.org

Ehlers-Danlos National Foundation
6399 Wilshire Blvd., Suite 510
Los Angeles, CA 90048
Phone: 323-651-3038
Fax: 323-651-1366
Web site: www.ednf.org
E-mail: loosejoint@aol.com

Fibromyalgia Association—USA
P.O. Box 20408
Columbus, OH 43220
Web site: www.fibromyalgiaassnusa.org
E-mail: USA.Fibromyalgia.Association@juno.com

Fibromyalgia Network
P.O. Box 31750
Tucson, Arizona 85751-1750
Phone: 520-290-5508
Web site: www.fmnetnews.com
E-mail: fmnetter@msn.com

The Hip Society
c/o Karen Anderson
951 Old County Road
Belmont, CA 94002
Phone: 650-956-6190
Fax: 650-508-2039

Lupus Foundation of America, Inc.
1300 Piccard Drive, Suite 200
Rockville, Maryland 20850
Phone: 301-670-9292
Fax: 301-670-9486
Toll free: 888-385-8787
Web site: www.lupus.org/lupus/
E-mail: lupuslfa@mail.erols.com

Lupus Foundation of America
Suite 123
260 Maple Court
Ventura, California 93033
Phone: 805-339-0443

National Institutes of Health (NAMSIC)
1 AMS Circle
Bethesda, MD 20892-3675
Phone: 301-495-4484
Fax: 301-587-4352
Web site: www.nih.gov/niams
Fast facts: 301-881-2731, information 24hr/
day by Fax

National Center for Complimentary
and Alternative Medicine Clearinghouse
P.O. Box 8218
Silver Spring, MD 20907-8218
Toll free: 888-644-6226
Fax: 301-495-4957
Web site: http://altmed.od.nih.gov/nccam/

National Certification Commission for
Acupuncturists
P.O. Box 97075
Washington, DC 20090-7075
Phone: 202-232-1404

National Chronic Pain Outreach Association, Inc.
P.O. Box 274
Millboro, VA 24460
Phone: 540-862-9437
Fax: 540-862-9486
Web site currently under construction: www.
chronicpain.org
E-mail: hcpoa@cfw.com

National Institute of Arthritis, Musculoskeletal and
Skin Diseases (NIAMS) Information Clearinghouse
Box AMS
9000 Rockville Pike
Bethesda, MD 20892
Phone: 301-495-4484
Web site: http://www.nih.gov/niams/

National Organization for Rare Disorders (NORD)
P.O. Box 8923
New Fairfield, CT 06812
Phone: 203-746-6518
Toll free: 800-999-6673
Fax: 203-746-6481
Web site: www.rarediseases.org
E-mail:orphan@rarediseases.org

The National Osteoporosis Foundation
1150 17th Street, NW
Washington, DC 20036-4603
Web site: www.nof.org

The National Psoriasis Foundation
6600 SW 92nd Avenue, Suite 300
Portland, OR 97223
Phone: (503) 244-7404
Fax: (503) 245-0626Fax

The Osteoporosis and Related Bone Diseases
National Resource Center
Toll free: 800-624-BONE

PACE Catalog Center
Arthritis Foundation Distribution Center
P.O. Box 1616
Alpahretta, GA 30009
Phone: 800-207-8633
Fax: 770-442-9742
Web site: www.arthritis.org

The Paget Foundation
Suite 1602
120 Wall Street
New York, NY 10005
Phone: 212-509-5335
Toll free: 800-23PAGET
Fax: 212-509-8492
Web site: www.paget.org
E-mail: pagetfdn@aol.com

Scleroderma Foundation
Suite 201
89 Newbury Street
Danvers, MA 01923
Phone: 978-750-4499
Toll free: 800-722-HOPE
Fax: 978-750-9902
Web site: www.scleroderma.org
E-mail: sclerofed@aol.com

Spondylitis Association of America (SAA)
14827 Ventura Blvd., Suite 222
P.O. Box 5872
Sherman Oaks, CA 91413
Phone: 818-981-1616
Toll free: 800-777-8189
Fax: 818-981-9826
Web site: www.spondylitis.org
E-mail: info@spondylitis.org

Traditional Acupuncture Institute
American City Building, Suite 100
10227 Wincopin Circle
Columbia, MD 21044-3422
Phone: 301-596-3675

Internet Resources
Food and Nutrition Information Center
http://www.nalusda.gov/fnic

The Mining Company
(This is a great source of information updated regularly on many health topics, with an extensive section on arthritis.)
http://www.arthritis.miningco.com

Arthritis Net
http://www.arthritisnet.com

Magazines
Arthritis Today
1330 West Peachtree Street
Atlanta, GA 30309
Toll free: 800-933-0032

Catalogs
Sammons Preston Enrichments; P.O. Box 5071, Bolingbrook, IL 50440-5071; 1-800-323-5547; Web site: www.sammonspreston.com

Independent Living Aids, Inc. Can-Do(TM) Products for your active independent life; 27 East Mall, Plainview, NY 11803; 1-800-537-2118

Functional Solutions, distributed by Access to Recreation, Inc.; 2509 E. Thousand Oaks Blvd., Suite 430, Thousand Oaks, CA 91362; 800-634-4351.

Don Krebs' Access to Recreation: Adaptive Recreation Equipment; P.O. Box 5072-430, Thousand Oaks, CA 91359-5072; 800-634-4351.

adaptAbility: Products for Quality Living; 75 Mill St., P.O. Box 515, Colchester, CT 06415-0515; 800-288-9941; E-mail: snswwide.com; Web site: www.snswwide.com.

S&S Opportunities, (geared more to therapists); P.O. Box 513, Colchester, CT 06415-0513; 800-266-8856; E-mail: service@snswwide.com; Web site: www.snswwide.com

S&S Healthcare; P.O. Box 513, Colchester, CT 06415-0513; 800-243-9232; E-mail: service@snswwide.com; Web site: www.snswwide.com

MaxiAids: Aids & Appliances for Independent Living; P.O. Box 3209, Farmingdale, NY 11735; 516-752-0521, 800-522-6294 (to order); E-mail: sales@maxiaids.com.

For more free information on assistive devices, visit the Web site of the American Association of Retired Persons (AARP) at http://www.aarp.com.

Legal resources and advocacies

CENTER FOR PATIENT ADVOCACY
Suite 108
1350 Beverly Road
McLean, VA 22101
Phone: 703/748-0400
Toll free: 800-846-7444
Web site: http://www.patientadvocacy.org/main/index.html
E-mail: patientadv@aol.com

FAMILIES USA
1334 G St. NW
Washington, DC 20005
Phone: 202-628-3030
Fax: 202-347-2417
http://www.familiesusa.org
E-mail: info@familiesusa.org

Families USA is a national nonprofit, nonpartisan organization dedicated to the achievement of high-quality, affordable health and long-term care for all Americans. Among other things, the organization manages a grassroots advocates' network of groups and individuals working for the consumer perspective in the national and state health policy debates, acts as a watchdog over government actions affecting health care, and produces health policy reports.

HANDSNET
Suite 375
2 North Second Street
San Jose, CA 95113
Phone: 408-291-5111
Fax: 408-291-5119
E-mail: http://www.handsnet.org/handsnet/
E-mail: HNINFO@handsnet.org

Founded in 1987, HandsNet links some 5,000 public interest and human-service organizations across the United States. Network members include national clearinghouses and research centers, community-based service providers, foundations, government agencies, public-policy advocates, legal services programs, and grassroots coalitions.

INSTITUTE FOR CHILD HEALTH POLICY
5700 SW 34th Street, Suite 323
Gainesville, FL 32608-5367
Phone: 352-392-5904
Toll free: 888-433-1851
Fax: 352-392-8822
Web site: http://www.ichp.ufl.edu/
E-mail: info@ichp.edu

The Institute focuses its attention on children in managed care with special emphasis on children with special health-care needs. Issues of access, cost, quality, and family involvement are principal areas of interest for their policy and program development, health-services research, and evaluation programs.

NATIONAL BIPARTISAN COMMISSION ON THE FUTURE OF MEDICARE
Adams Building, Library of Congress
101 Independence Ave., SE
Washington, DC 20540-1998
Web site: http://medicare.commission.gov/
medicare/index.html

The National Bipartisan Commission on the Future of Medicare was created by Congress in the Balanced Budget Act of 1997. Under that act, the Commission is charged with examining the

Medicare program and making recommendations to strengthen and improve it in time for the retirement of the "Baby Boomers." The Commission's work will be open to the public, and the members will seek ways to keep you informed and involved.

NATIONAL COALITION ON HEALTH CARE

555 13th St. NW
Washington, DC 20004
Phone: 202-637-6830
Fax: 202-347-2417
Web site: http://www.americashealth.org/
E-mail: info@nchc.org

The National Coalition on Health Care is the nation's largest and most broadly representative alliance working to improve America's health care. Rigorously nonpartisan, the Coalition is comprised of almost 100 groups, representing large and small businesses, labor unions, consumer groups, religious groups, and primary care providers. The coalition members support the following principles:

- Securing health insurance for all.
- Improved quality of care.
- Cost containment.
- Equitable financing.
- Simplified administration.

NATIONAL COUNCIL ON AGING

Phone: 202-479-6606 Extn. 6605
Fax: 202-479-0735
Web site: http://scooby.mrl.nyu.edu:8000/
E-mail: mbrsvcs@ncoa.org

As an association of more than 7,500 members—organizations and individuals—who work with, for, and on behalf of older persons, NCOA is open for membership to those who share our commitment "to promoting the dignity, self-determination, well-being, and contributions of older persons and to enhancing the field of aging through leadership, service, education, and advocacy."

NATIONAL SENIOR CITIZENS LAW CENTER
Suite 400
1101 14th St., NW
Washington, DC 20005
Phone: 202-289-6976
Fax: 202-289-7224
Web site: http://www.nsclc.org/
E-mail: nsclc@nsclc.org

The National Senior Citizens Law Center was established in 1972 to help older individuals live their lives in dignity and freedom from poverty, through legal work in support of elderly poor clients, client groups, and Elder Law attorneys. NSCLC attorneys are knowledgeable in a broad range of legal issues and practice areas that affect the security and welfare of older persons of limited income.

PUBLIC CITIZEN HEALTH RESEARCH GROUP
http://www.citizen.org/hrg/
E-mail: public_citizen@citizen.org

Founded by Ralph Nader in 1971, Public Citizen is the consumer's eyes and ears in Washington. Its Health Research Group fights for safe foods, drugs, and medical devices; for greater consumer control over personal health decisions; and for universal access to quality health care.

THE ROBERT WOOD JOHNSON FOUNDATION
P.O. Box 2316
Princeton, NJ 08543-2316
Phone: 609-452-8701
Web site: http://www.rwjf.org/main.html
E-mail: mail@rwjf.org

The Robert Wood Johnson Foundation is the nation's largest philanthropy devoted exclusively to health and health care. The Foundation concentrates its grant making in three goal areas: to assure that all Americans have access to basic health care at reasonable cost; to improve the way services are organized and provided to people with chronic health conditions; and to reduce the personal, social, and economic harm caused by substance abuse—tobacco, alcohol, and illicit drugs.

Recommended Reading

Shelley Peterman Schwarz, *250 Tips for Making Life with Arthritis Easier.* Longstreet Press, 1997.

Roberta Larson Duyff, M.S., *The American Dietetic Association's Complete Food & Nutrition Guide.* Chronimed Publishing, 1996.

Denise Lang, *Coping with Lyme Disease: A Practical Guide to Dealing with Diagnosis and Treatment.* Henry Holt, 1997.

Miryam Ehrlich Williamson, *The Fibromyalgia Relief Book: 213 Ideas for Improving Your Quality of Life.* Walker & Co, 1998.

Sheldon Paul Blau, M.D. with Dodi Schultz, *Living with Lupus.* Addison-Wesley, 1993

Michael Castleman, *Nature's Cure.* Rodale Press, 1997.

Virginia Tortorica Aldape, *Nicole's Story: A Book About a Girl with Juvenile Rheumatoid Arthritis by Reading Level: Ages 4–8.* Lerner Publications Company, 1996.

Nancy L. Clouse, *Pink Paper Swans by Reading Level: Ages 4–8*. Wm. B. Eeerdmans Publishing Co., 1994.

Debra Fulgham Bruce, *The Unofficial Guide to Alternative Medicine*. Macmillan, 1997.

Miriam E. Nelson, PhD, with Sarah Wernick, *Strong Women Stay Young*. Bantam, 1997.

Miriam E. Nelson, PhD, with Sarah Wernick, *Strong Women Stay Slim*. Bantam, 1998

A

The *Unofficial Guide*™ Reader Questionnaire

If you would like to express your opinion about arthritis or this guide, please complete this questionnaire and mail it to:

The *Unofficial Guide*™ Reader Questionnaire
Macmillan Lifestyle Group
1633 Broadway, floor 7
New York, NY 10019-6785

Gender: ___ M ___ F

Age: ___ Under 30 ___ 31–40 ___ 41–50
___ Over 50

Education: ___ High school ___ College
___ Graduate/Professional

What is your occupation?

_____

How did you hear about this guide?
___ Friend or relative
___ Newspaper, magazine, or Internet
___ Radio or TV
___ Recommended at bookstore
___ Recommended by librarian
___ Picked it up on my own
___ Familiar with the *Unofficial Guide*™ travel series

Did you go to the bookstore specifically for a book on arthritis? Yes ___ No ___

Have you used any other Unofficial Guides™ *?*
Yes ___ No ___

If Yes, which ones?

_____
_____
_____

What other book(s) on arthritis have you pur-chased?

_____

_____

_____

Was this book:
___ more helpful than other(s)
___ less helpful than other(s)

Do you think this book was worth its price?
Yes ___   No ___

Did this book cover all topics related to arthritis adequately?
Yes ___   No ___

Please explain your answer:

_____

_____

_____

Were there any specific sections in this book that were of particular help to you?   Yes ___   No ___

Please explain your answer:

_____

_____

_____

On a scale of 1 to 10, with 10 being the best rat-ing, how would you rate this guide? ___

What other titles would you like to see published in the Unofficial Guide™ series?

_____

_____

Are Unofficial Guides™ readily available in your area?   Yes ___   No ___

Other comments:

_____

_____

_____

_____

Get the inside scoop...with the *Unofficial Guides™!*

The Unofficial Guide to Acing the Interview
   ISBN: 0-02-862924-8 Price: $15.95

The Unofficial Guide to Alternative Medicine
   ISBN: 0-02-862526-9 Price: $15.95

The Unofficial Guide to Buying or Leasing a Car
   ISBN: 0-02-862524-2 Price: $15.95

The Unofficial Guide to Buying a Home
   ISBN: 0-02-862461-0 Price: $15.95

The Unofficial Guide to Childcare
   ISBN: 0-02-862457-2 Price: $15.95

The Unofficial Guide to Cosmetic Surgery
   ISBN: 0-02-862522-6 Price: $15.95

The Unofficial Guide to Dieting Safely
   ISBN: 0-02-862521-8 Price: $15.95

The Unofficial Guide to Divorce
   ISBN: 0-02-862455-6 Price: $15.95

The Unofficial Guide to Earning What You Deserve
   ISBN: 0-02-862716-4 Price: $15.95

The Unofficial Guide to Hiring and Firing People
   ISBN: 0-02-862523-4 Price: $15.95

The Unofficial Guide to Hiring Contractors
   ISBN: 0-02-862460-2 Price: $15.95

The *Unofficial Guide to Having a Baby*
   ISBN: 0-02-862695-8   Price: $15.95

The Unofficial Guide to Investing
   ISBN: 0-02-862458-0 Price: $15.95

The Unofficial Guide to Planning Your Wedding
   ISBN: 0-02-862459-9 Price: $15.95

All books in the *Unofficial Guide™* series are available at your local bookseller, or by calling 1-800-428-5331.

About the Authors

Lisa Iannucci and Dr. Mark Horowitz can tell you everything you need to know about arthritis. Lisa Iannucci has been researching and writing in the field of health for the last decade. Her articles have been published in *American Health, Muscle and Fitness, Energy Times, Weight Watchers,* and *FDA Consumer* magazines. She has also published on health related topics in *Practical Homeowner* on remodeling your home during pregnancy and in *Parenting Magazine.* She has also published for medical trade journals and newsletters, including *Ocular Surgery News* and *Rehab Management,* and is the author of *Birth Defects* (Enslo Publishing, 1999), a reference book for elementary school children. Her recent research has led her to writing articles on lead poisoning and the "sick building syndrome."

Ms. Iannucci lives with her husband, Jeff, and her three children, Nicole, Travis, and Samantha, in upstate New York. She teaches writing at Duchess Community College and Ulster Community College.

Dr. Mark Horowitz is a co-author of *Living With Lupus: A Comprehensive Guide to Understanding and Controlling Lupus While Getting on With Your Life* (Plume, 1994). Dr. Horowitz is affiliated with the Mount Sinai Hospital in New York, where he specializes in rheumatology and his clinical interests include systemic lupus and osteoporosis. Dr. Horowitz graduated from Northeastern Ohio Universities College of Medicine, and held a residency at Mount Sinai Medical Center.